Introduction to Medical Mycology

Glenn S. Bulmer, Ph.D.

Professor (Medical Mycology)
Department of Microbiology and Immunology
University of Oklahoma Health Sciences Center

YEAR BOOK MEDICAL PUBLISHERS, INC.

CHICAGO • LONDON

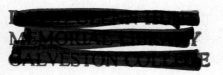

Dedication: MAHAL

Library of Congress Cataloging in Publication Data

Bulmer, Glenn S
  Introduction to medical mycology.

  Editions for 1967 – 1969 published under title: Lectures in medical mycology.
  Includes index.
  1. Medical mycology.   I. Title.
RC117.B84   616.01'5   79-14007
ISBN 0-8151-1320-X

Preface

THIS BOOK is designed for persons who are interested in an introduction to the most important pathogenic fungi. The material is intentionally abbreviated and simplified in the hope that this will stimulate the reader to delve further into study of the mycoses.

Since 1962, I have presented all of the fungus disease lectures at the University of Oklahoma Health Sciences Center to medical, graduate and paramedical students. Because most of these students have never been exposed to any aspect of mycology, I have found it best to begin with a general introduction to the fungi and then present the mycoses in a straightforward and highly structured fashion. This book grew out of my *Lectures in Medical Mycology,* which I produced locally. It includes an introductory chapter on medical mycology, seven chapters on various mycoses, figures, black and white reproductions of all of the 35mm slides available in a complementary set, a commentary on each of the slides, self-evaluation questions at the end of each chapter and a final self-evaluation exercise which covers all of the material included in this book.

A set of 332 35mm color slides is available as an accompaniment to the book. It is intended for instructors who lecture on medical mycology, for libraries, and for clinical and microbiology departments. Representing more than 15 years of collecting and photographing medical mycology material, the slide set forms an important complement to the text.

I would like to thank Glenn Roberts, Ph.D., at the Mayo Clinic and Betty Russell, M.S., at the Stanford University Medical Center for their helpful comments and suggestions, many of which have been incorporated in this book.

GLENN S. BULMER

Special Acknowledgment

I am especially grateful to Mui-Quy-Bong, M.D., M.P.H., T.M., whose excellent illustrations have contributed so greatly to the book.

Contents

1 / Introduction to Medical Mycology

DEFINITION

FUNGI ARE AEROBIC, nucleated, achlorophyllous organisms, which typically reproduce sexually and/or asexually. These organisms' usually filamentous branched somatic structures are surrounded by a true cell wall. The following terms in this definition deserve further emphasis:

Aerobic. All true fungi are aerobic.

Nucleated. This term is included in the definition in an attempt to differentiate fungi from bacteria. Although bacteria have nuclear material, it is not organized into chromosomes, and a nuclear membrane is lacking. In contrast, the nuclei of fungi are similar to the nuclei found in mammalian cells.

Achlorophyllous. This means that fungi lack chlorophyll and implies that most of them are saprophytic.

Sexual and/or asexual reproduction. Many fungi reproduce by both sexual (meiosis) and asexual (mitosis) means. This is particularly important in establishing the taxonomy of fungi.

Cell wall. The presence of a true cell wall places fungi in the plant kingdom. In many instances the cell walls contain large amounts of chitin.

There are more than 100,000 species of fungi. They exhibit great variation in size, morphology, mode of reproduction and methods of dissemination. Some fungi are as small as 3 microns whereas others exceed 3 feet in diameter.

REPRODUCTION OF FUNGI

YEASTS. — All yeasts are fungi. Most are single-celled structures with a thick cell wall. A yeast cell is a distinct entity, i.e., it is a single plant. Yeasts usually multiply asexually by budding. A bud is sometimes called a blastospore. This process of budding is mitotic and results in the production of two cells (Fig. 1–1).

HYPHAE. — Hyphae are long, slender, branching tubes, generally 3 to 10 microns in diameter. If hyphae have crosswalls, the fungus is said to be septate. If crosswalls are not present, the fungus is said to be coenocytic or nonseptate (Fig. 1–2). The presence or absence of these crosswalls can be a morphological aid in distinguishing between certain etiologic agents of specific mycoses. Hyphae might be considered as being the root system of most fungi. A mass of hyphae is called mycelium(ia).

SPORES. — Spores are functionally similar to the seeds of higher plants. There are two types of spores: sexual and asexual. If the spores are produced sexually, the mechanism is the same as sexual reproduction in all forms of life. Sexual reproduction may be defined as an alternation between karyogamy

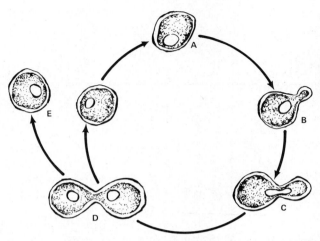

Fig 1–1.—A yeast reproducing. **A,** yeast cell. **B,** yeast cell with bud. **C,** bud enlarged. **D,** bud enlarges further and eventually breaks off. **E,** two yeast cells.

and meiosis. Karyogamy is nuclear fusion. Meiosis is reduction division, with a diploid nucleus giving rise to four haploid products.

Asexual reproduction occurs strictly by the process of mitosis. This is the most common process by which spores are produced in fungi. The manner in which spores are produced is important in the identification of fungi. Some spores, for example, are borne in a sac-like structure called a sporangium. The spores thus contained are sporangiospores. Other spores, which are produced on the tips or sides of hyphae, are called conidia (conidium)*; conidia may vary in size, shape and color (Fig. 1–3). They may be formed in chains or clumps and may be multi- or single-celled (Fig. 1–4).

In some fungi the hyphal cells may become specialized spores. If a cell enlarges and develops thick walls, it is called a chlamydospore. In *Geotri-*

---

*Technically, a conidium is produced on a specialized structure called a conidio-phore (Fig 1–4, *A* and *D*). A spore which is produced directly on a hypha or a hyphal tip is called an aleuriospore. When a fungus produces two sizes of aleuriospores, the larger one is called a macroaleuriospore, and the smaller one is called a microaleurio-spore.

Fig 1–2.—Fungal hyphae. **A,** coenocytic hypha. **B,** septate hypha. **C,** septum.

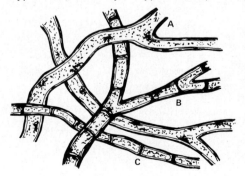

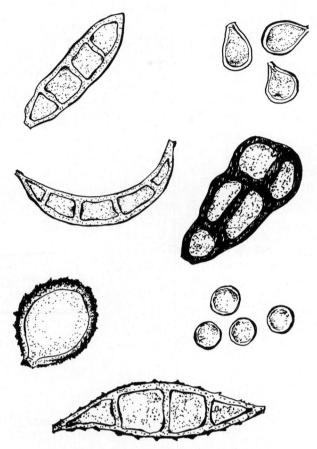

Fig 1–3. — A few examples of fungal spores.

chum candidum the hyphal cells separate from one another to form flat-ended asexual spores known as oidia(ium). In *Coccidioides immitis,* the hyphal cells break apart (much as they do in the formation of oidia): these are called arthrospores (Fig. 1–5). Fragmentation may occur naturally by the action of wind, soil movement or insects.

The great variation in spore morphology and the manner in which spores are produced provide the major means for identifying fungi.

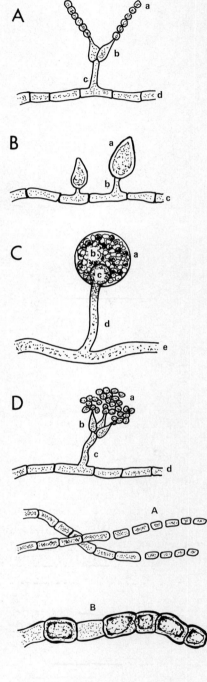

Fig 1–4.—Various ways that fungal spores are borne. **A,** conidia produced in chains—*a,* conidia in a chain; *b,* sterigma; *c,* conidiophore; *d,* septate hypha. **B,** conidia borne singly—*a,* single-celled conidium; *b,* conidiophore; *c,* septate hypha. **C,** spores produced in sporangium—*a,* sporangium; *b,* sporangiospores; *c,* columella; *d,* sporangiophore; *e,* coenocytic hypha. **D,** conidia in a clump—*a,* conidia in a clump; *b,* several sterigmata; *c,* conidiophore; *d,* septate hypha.

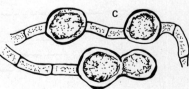

Fig 1–5.—Other types of fungal spores. **A,** oidia. **B,** arthrospores. **C,** chlamydospores.

Slides

The following slides illustrate some of the points previously mentioned.

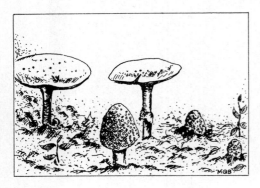

Slide 1–1.—These are mushrooms, which most people consider to be representative of a typical fungus. There is no easy or clearcut way of distinguishing between a mushroom and a toadstool. Old wives' tales say that poisonous mushrooms turn the color of a silver spoon or a copper coin when boiled and that it is easy to peel the top skin off an edible mushroom. None of these is true. The only truly certain way to determine whether a fungus is a mushroom or a toadstool is to have the specific organism in question identified by a mycologist.

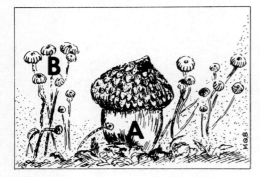

Slide 1–2.—These field mushrooms are about an inch high. This slide merely illustrates the great variation in size seen among mushrooms. In the center of this photograph (A) is an acorn from an oak tree: the small, white, flower-like structures around the acorn are the caps of the mushrooms (B).

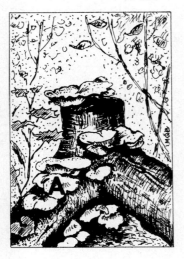

Slide 1–3.—This is another type of fungus, the so-called oyster mushroom (A). As with so many other mushrooms, what is visible is the smallest part of the fungus. The white caps growing on the log are the fruiting structures whose sole purpose is to bear spores. The greater part of this organism is the mycelial system located inside the tree.

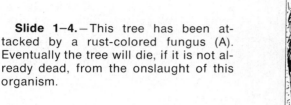

Slide 1–4.—This tree has been attacked by a rust-colored fungus (A). Eventually the tree will die, if it is not already dead, from the onslaught of this organism.

Slide 1–5.—Technically speaking, mushrooms belong to a class of fungi known as Basidiomycetes. If one were to section the gill-like structures on the underside of a mushroom cap and examine them under the microscope, one would see structures as indicated in this slide. In the middle, two spherical spores (A) are attached to a larger cell (B). The larger cell is known as a basidium. Within the basidium, meiosis has occurred, and the end products, haploid nuclei, migrate out into the spores (A).

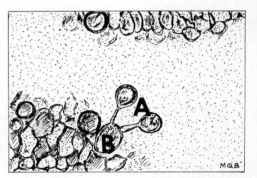

Slide 1–6.—In the world of microbiology, this is the manner in which fungi are usually seen. Two plates of media were exposed to the air for 10 minutes—both at the same site. On both of the plates are dozens of fungal colonies growing on each medium. The individual colonies differ in size, shape and color. Each one of the colonies arose from airborne spores which landed on the medium during the exposure period and then developed into a characteristic colony. The medium in the plate which contains the smaller colonies (A) is similar to the medium in the other plate, except that it contains (1) cycloheximide, an antibiotic which inhibits the growth of many of the so-called contaminating or airborne fungi and (2) chloramphenicol, an antibiotic which inhibits the growth of many bacteria. This medium is used frequently in medical mycology because the antibiotics usually do not inhibit the growth of human fungal pathogens.

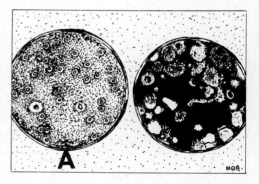

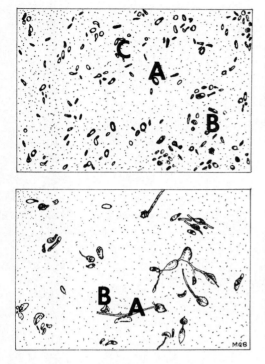

Slide 1–7.—This is a photomicrograph of a typical yeast. In this slide are several dozen yeast cells. Some are round (A); others are somewhat elongated (B). Small buds (blastospores) project out of the side of some of the cells (C).

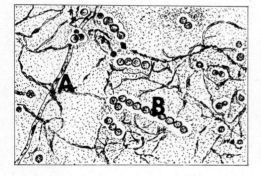

Slide 1–8.—This is another type of yeast—merely to illustrate that yeasts may have somewhat differing morphologies. This yeast, known as *Sporobolomyces,* is not a human pathogen. When these cells bud, they first produce long, slender projections (A). At the end of these projections the bud is formed (B).

The next several slides are examples of hyphae and show the way that filamentous fungi form spores. Fungi are identified by the different morphological forms.

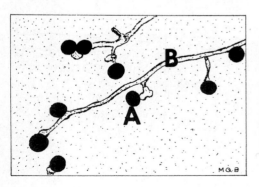

Slide 1–9.—This organism is called *Scopulariopsis.* It is a fungus which forms septate hyphae that can be seen in the background on this slide (A). Hyphae are the darker, slender, long tubes. In the foreground of this photomicrograph are several long chains of spores (B). These spores are approximately 5 microns in diameter, have a rough surface and are spherical. In this case, they appear to be surrounded by a clear halo, a photographic artifact resulting from the use of phase photography.

Slide 1–10.—This is an organism known as *Nigrospora,* which means "black spore." The 9 jet black structures in this photomicrograph are the single-celled spores (A). Each spore is approximately 15 microns in diameter. The long, slender, almost clear tubes are the septate hyphae (B).

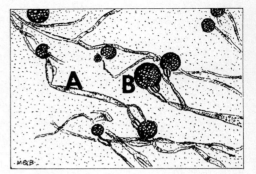

Slide 1–11.—This organism is called *Gliocladium*. Arising from the clear hyphae (A) are the spore-bearing structures. The large, dark masses contain from 30 to 50 small spores (B). This is an example of how some fungi produce their spores in clumps.

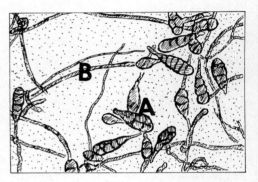

Slide 1–12.—This is the plant pathogen *Alternaria*. Hand-grenade-shaped structures in this photomicrograph are the large spores of this fungus (A). Each spore is approximately 20 to 40 microns and brown (dematiaceous) in color. Note that each spore has many horizontal and longitudinal septa. Also note the septate, dematiaceous hyphae (B).

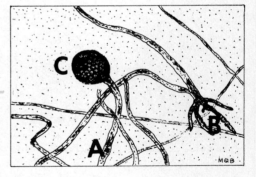

Slide 1–13.—This organism, known as *Rhizopus,* is characterized by coenocytic hyphae (A), the formation of root-like structures called rhizoids (B) and the dark spherical structure known as a sporangium (C). A mature sporangium may contain up to 100 sporangiospores.

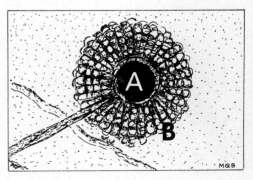

Slide 1–14.—This organism is *Syncephalastrum,* another fungus which produces its spores in sporangia. However, for this organism sporangium formation is different. Surrounding the very dark central structure (A) are numerous small, almost clear projections (B). Each of these individual structures is a sporangium, and each contains from 3 to 5 sporangiospores.

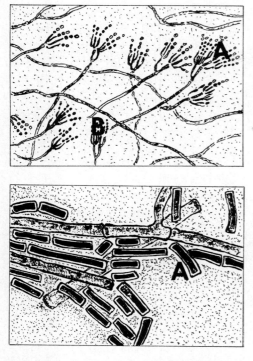

Slide 1–15.—This is *Penicillium,* the organism which produces penicillin. The spores of *Penicillium* are very small, i.e., 3 to 5 microns. They are borne in long chains, thus giving the appearance of a brush (A, B).

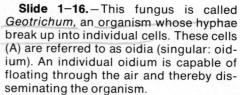

Slide 1–16.—This fungus is called *Geotrichum,* an organism whose hyphae break up into individual cells. These cells (A) are referred to as oidia (singular: oidium). An individual oidium is capable of floating through the air and thereby disseminating the organism.

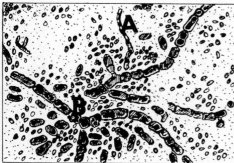

Slide 1–17.—This is an organism called *Aureobasidium.* An older term, *Pullularia,* is still used in several textbooks. It is characterized by the presence of clear hyphae (A) *and* dark brown (dematiaceous) hyphae (B).

In most mycology slides, although the hyphae are described as clear, they are visualized as being blue. The hyphae look blue because the organism was suspended in a mounting fluid, lactophenol cotton blue.

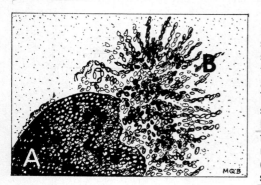

Slide 1–18.—The dark (brown or dematiaceous) body (A) in this picture is a spore sac, called an ascocarp. Unlike a sporangium, this is a much larger structure, i.e., 300 to 500 microns in diameter, and it has a very tough, thick outer wall. This is the structure in which sexual spores are produced for fungi which belong to the class Ascomycetes. Exuding from this large, fruiting structure are many long, slender, sac-like structures (B), which are asci (singular: ascus). Inside each ascus are 4 or 8 ascospores.

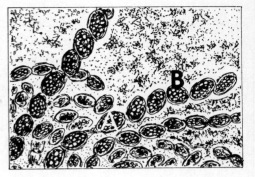

Slide 1–19.—This is a higher magnification of Slide 1–18. Ascospores (A) are held in an ascus by a very fine membrane (B). Because ascospores arise from meiosis, there are usually 4 or 8 in each ascus.

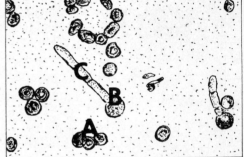

Slide 1–20.—This slide shows a number of smooth-walled, spherical, dematiacious spores. Some of these spores appear to be collapsed (A), probably owing to desiccation. The important feature of this slide is that it shows the process known as spore germination. Note that the one spore in the middle of the slide (B) has a long, slender, septate tube (C) coming out of it. This is referred to as a "germ tube," although it actually is a septate hypha. Close observation shows that one other spore in this slide has begun to germinate. The process of spore germination is very similar in all of the fungi, although some organisms may produce more than one germ tube from a single spore.

THE FUNGAL CELL

The fungal cell is very similar in many ways to the cells found in higher forms of life. Septate fungi are septate only from a morphological point of view. Physiologically, they are coenocytic because the septa have pores in them large enough to allow nuclei to pass through. One outstanding characteristic of fungal cells is that they have very thick cell walls. Inside the cell wall is a plasma membrane. Every fungal cell contains one or more nuclei with true chromosomes. These chromosomes function in the same manner as do the chromosomes in all forms of higher life. The nuclei of fungi are usually haploid but some fungi, although retaining the haploid state, have many nuclei within a cell. Fungal cells have an endoplasmic reticulum, many fat storage depots and mitochondria.

The cell wall generally contains only 5–10% protein. In the cell walls of yeasts, the major components are carbohydrate polymers, such as glucans and mannans, which usually constitute 50–60% of the cell wall. The cell wall of filamentous fungi generally has a very high content of chitin. Chitin, made of N-acetyl glucosamine, is one of the toughest biologically produced materials.

WHERE ARE FUNGI FOUND?

Fungi are found everywhere. They are ubiquitous. They are even found in sea water and in the arctic ice. There is no escaping from fungi.

MEDICAL MYCOLOGY

Why is it important to consider fungi as etiologic agents of disease? A few years ago, it was merely of academic interest to be able to diagnose a fungus disease. In the past few years, however, several antibiotics have been developed that are quite effective in treating mycotic infections. Many of the cutaneous and systemic mycoses can now be cured. For this reason, diagnosis of a specific fungal disease is now important. Accurate diagnosis of fungal diseases is essential in epidemiological matters, such as in delineating endemic areas for a disease and in attempting to control it. The number of mycoses being diagnosed has increased dramatically throughout the world. Many of the serious mycoses seen today probably begin, or are worsened, because the patient has another disease or is on immunosuppressive therapy. Therefore, the diagnosis of a specific mycosis may offer clues to a patient's other underlying problems.

Factors in Identifying a Mycotic Disease

1. In almost all cases, fungus diseases are chronic, i.e., slowly evolving diseases that take months or even years to develop. Major exceptions to this are the primary pulmonary form of histoplasmosis and coccidioidomycosis and an acute form of nocardiosis.
2. The history obtained from the patient can be important. Most of the fungi causing human disease grow in soil; therefore, many of the patients with mycoses have had contact with soil. Because some of the mycoses have well-defined endemic areas, it can be important to know where the patient was raised, has lived and worked and has traveled in recent years.
3. Such factors as diabetes, many types of cancers, alcoholism, recent surgery and administration of immunosuppressive agents and/or antibiotics predispose one to systemic mycoses.
4. Only one fungus disease, sporotrichosis, has a very clear-cut clinical picture. The clinical picture for cutaneous lymphatic sporotrichosis is almost completely diagnostic. In other cases, the clinical picture of the disease process is of little value in enabling one to diagnose a specific disease. At best, the clinical picture might lead one to suspect that a fungus is involved.
5. An important tool in the diagnosis of a fungus disease is the appearance of the organism in tissue. There are two methods of preparing tissue for fungal examination:

   Direct Examination. — The specimen (which may be from a biopsy, pus sample, sputum specimen or spinal fluid) is placed directly on a microscope slide. Generally, a drop or two of KOH (10–20%) is added. The KOH clears away much of the tissue debris but does not break down fungal structures, thus making it easier to see the fungus. The examiner adds a coverslip, presses it down and observes the specimen microscopically.

Stained Histology Slide.—Most fungi are larger than 3 microns, so it is much easier to see fungi than bacteria in stained slides. The most commonly used stains for observing fungi in tissue are the periodic acid-Schiff (PAS) and Gomori's methenamine silver (GMS).

Six Ways That Fungi May Be Observed in Tissue

YEAST CELLS.—One of the most common forms in which one sees fungi in tissue is yeast cells. The methenamine silver stain (GMS) is particularly valuable for visualizing yeast and other forms of fungi in tissue.

Yeast cells may be seen intracellularly; e.g., *Histoplasma capsulatum* is one of the few fungi that can be classified as an intracellular parasite.

In cryptococcosis, most yeast cells have a large distinguishing capsule.

Many yeast cells in tissue exhibit buds. A large neck (broad base) between the mother cell and the bud is a valuable diagnostic feature in cases of blastomycosis. Some yeast cells have multiple buds, e.g., the cause of paracoccidioidomycosis. The size of yeast cells is an important point, e.g., yeast cells of *H. capsulatum* are 3–5 microns, whereas cells of *Blastomyces dermatitidis* are 8–15 microns in diameter. The following are pictures of yeast cells.

Slides

Slide 1–21.—Here are 6 or 7 yeast cells growing in brain tissue. The individual cells (A) are approximately 10 microns in diameter. The outstanding feature of these yeast cells is that they are surrounded by a huge, clear capsule (B). *Cryptococcus neoformans* apparently is the only pathogenic encapsulated yeast.

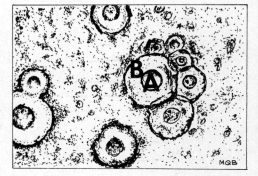

Slide 1–22.—Most of the yeast cells (A) seen in this slide are somewhat larger than the ones in Slide 1–21. However, the outstanding characteristic of these yeast cells is that they multiply by forming numerous very small buds (B). This organism is *Paracoccidioides (Blastomyces) brasiliensis,* which causes paracoccidioidomycosis.

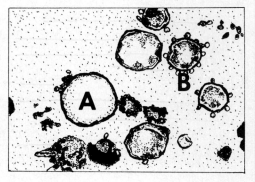

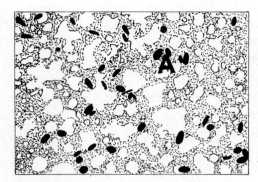

Slide 1–23.—This is a gram stain prepared from mouse tissue infected with *Sporothrix schenckii*. All of the darkly stained, gram-positive yeast cells (A) are the etiologic agent. The characteristic feature of the yeast cells of this pathogenic fungus is that many of them are long and slender and therefore are frequently described as being "cigar-like" in shape.

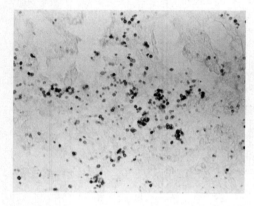

Slide 1–24.—This is a methenamine silver stain (GMS) from a person with histoplasmosis. The silver stain is an excellent method of visualizing fungi in tissue because all fungi take up silver. The main feature of these yeast cells is the fact that they are very small, i.e., 3–5 microns in diameter.

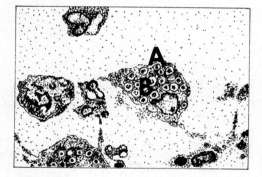

Slide 1–25.—Here again is *H. capsulatum*. However, this is a histopathology section through a node stained with hematoxylin and eosin (H&E). Note the cell nearly in the middle of the field (A). Inside this cell are numerous very small yeast cells (B). Close observation may give the impression that these yeast cells have a small halo, or capsule, around them. This erroneously led early investigators to believe that this organism was encapsulated, and to this day the species name of this organism is *capsulatum*. It is now known that the so-called capsule is a fixation artifact.

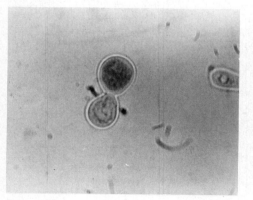

Slide 1–26.—This is yet another example of yeast cells. In this slide is a yeast cell in the process of division. The outstanding features of this cell are that it is 8–15 microns in diameter, and the bud being formed on the parent cell is attached with a broad-based neck. In contrast, when most yeast cells bud, the new cell is pinched off from the parent cell by a narrow neck. This broad-based neck and the size of the mature yeast cells are diagnostic for the organism *(Blastomyces dermatitidis),* which causes blastomycosis.

SPORANGIA. — Sporangia are large, sac-like structures which fill with spores as they mature. Some books refer to them as spherules. The spores contained in these sacs are called sporangiospores or endospores. The following slides show examples of sporangia.

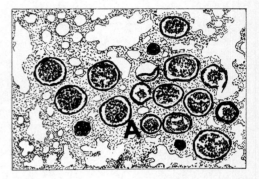

Slide 1–27. — All of the spherical, darkly stained structures (A) in the middle of this slide are sporangia (or "spherules"). This picture is from a case of rhinosporidiosis.

Slide 1–28. — In this slide is a single sporangium under higher magnification (A). This individual sporangium is more than 100 microns in diameter and has a thick cell wall. Inside it are numerous sporangiospores (B) or endospores. This, again, is rhinosporidiosis.

Slide 1–29. — This is a photomicrograph of an unstained preparation of tissue from an animal with coccidioidomycosis. In this preparation are a sporangium (spherule) (A) which contains numerous sporangiospores (endospores), and 2 larger sporangia (B) which have matured to the point where they have broken open and released their spores, thus appearing empty.

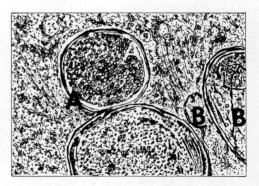

HYPHAE. — Hyphae can be coenocytic, septate, very fine, hyaline or dematiaceous. The following series of slides shows the types of hyphae that different fungi produce in tissue.

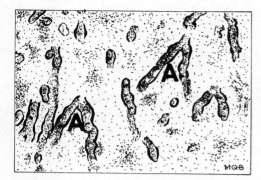

Slide 1-30.—These hyphae have a diameter of between 5 and 10 microns. The characteristic feature of these hyphae is the dichotomous branching (A). The associated disease is aspergillosis.

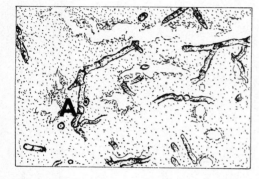

Slide 1-31.—The hyphae scattered throughout this tissue section are septate (A). This patient has aspergillosis.

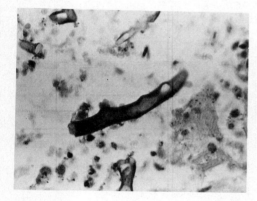

Slide 1-32.—In contrast to the hyphae in Slides 1-30 and 1-31, this hypha is larger, i.e., usually in excess of 10 microns in diameter, and is coenocytic. This is from a case of phycomycosis. Some medical mycologists now prefer the term "zygomycosis" for this disease.

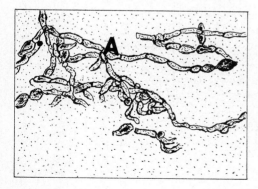

Slide 1-33.—This is an unstained preparation of pus from a brain abscess. Because of the brown color of the hyphae (A) in an unstained preparation, they are referred to as dematiacious. Several dematiacious fungi cause brain and subcutaneous abscesses. Some authors call this disease cladosporiosis or phaeohyphomycosis.

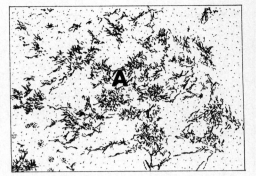

Slide 1–34.—This is a methenamine silver stain (GMS) of filaments as seen in a typical case of nocardiosis. Although it is difficult to visualize them clearly at this magnification, the outstanding feature of these filaments (A) is that they are extremely fine, i.e., approximately 1 micron or less in diameter.

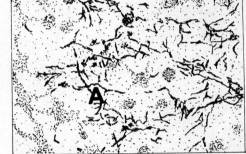

Slide 1–35.—This is a higher magnification of Slide 1–34. In this preparation, it is easier to see the very fine, delicate filaments which have a tendency to break into bacillary forms.

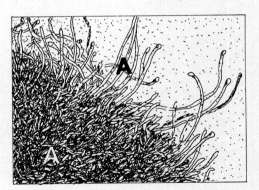

Slide 1–36.—This is a photomicrograph of tissue removed from a patient with mycotic keratitis. Note the abundance of nondematiaceous hyphae (A). Dermatophytic fungi, growing in skin or nails, give a similar appearance. In this case, the etiologic agent was a species of *Fusarium.*

GRANULES.—Granules are tightly packed masses of hyphae or filaments which are surrounded by a tough outer rind. Granules may be grossly visible, 0.5–10 mm in diameter. Microscopically, they contain either fine and delicate filaments or thick and septate hyphae. Examples of granules are in the next slides.

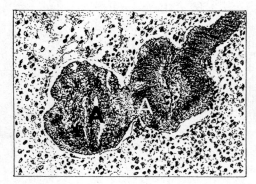

Slide 1–37.—This is an "actinomycotic granule." The granule is the large, lobulated structure (red-stained) which takes up almost the entire photograph (A).

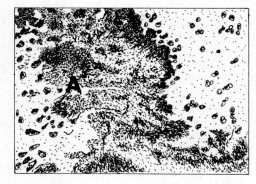

Slide 1–38.—This is a higher magnification of a granule similar to the one seen in Slide 1–37. The granule is composed of very fine, delicately branched filaments (A) which are less than 1 micron in diameter. This is from a case of actinomycosis.

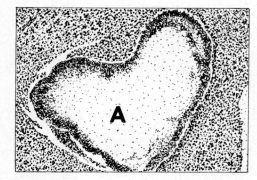

Slide 1–39.—This is another type of granule, the type seen in cases of eumycotic (true fungi) mycetoma. Granules in this disease (A) are relatively large and are surrounded by a very thick rind which may be variously colored. This is from a case of madura foot (mycetoma) or maduromycosis.

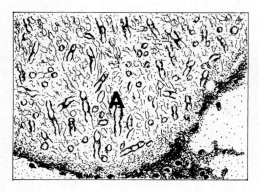

Slide 1–40.—This is a higher magnification of a granule from a case of eumycotic mycetoma. The entire structure seen in the picture is a granule. The inside of the granule is composed of numerous strands of hyphae (A) which are approximately 5 microns in diameter.

FISSION BODIES.—Fission bodies are spherical, dematiaceous structures which neither bud nor produce hyphae; division is by splitting down the middle (i.e., fission). Some medical mycologists prefer to call these structures "sclerotic bodies."

Slide 1–41.—In this photomicrograph is an example of fission *(sclerotic)* bodies. These structures are characteristic of the disease known as chromomycosis. There are two such structures in this slide (A, B). The most obvious fission body (A) is almost in the middle of the field; it is dematiaceous, does not have any buds and appears to be dividing by fission.

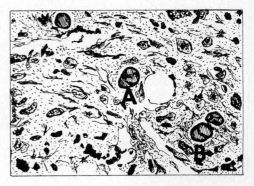

COMBINATION OF YEAST CELLS AND HYPHAE.—This is seen in candidiasis only.

Slide 1–42.—This is the organism *Candida albicans,* seen growing on a laboratory identification medium (chlamydospore agar). In this slide are 3 forms of the fungus: The dark (blue), spherical structures are known as chlamydospores (A); scattered all over the field and less darkly stained than the chlamydospores are hundreds of small yeast cells (B) and occasional pseudo-hyphae (C). To identify this organism in the laboratory, look for all three of these structures. When this organism grows in vivo, look for the combination of yeast cells and hyphae only; no chlamydospores are present.

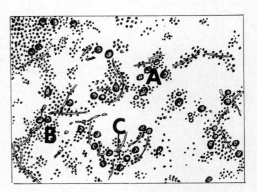

Slide 1–43.—This is a gram stain of sputum from a debilitated patient with pulmonary candidiasis. Note the abundant gram-positive hyphae (A). Additionally, one can see a few yeast cells (B). In sputum, the overabundance of hyphae with very few yeast cells often indicates pulmonary (not oral) involvement.

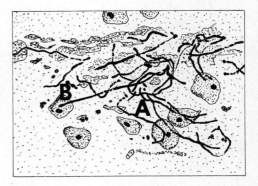

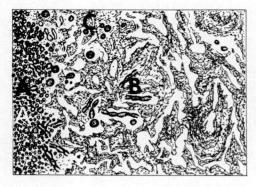

Slide 1–44.—This is a methenamine silver stain (GMS) of a kidney section from a patient with candidiasis. All of the black-stained bodies in this slide are the organism *Candida albicans* (A). In this section, the organism is producing hyphae (B) and yeast cells (C).

GENERAL FEATURES OF CULTURING FUNGI

1. Almost all animal pathogens are extremely slow-growing. It may take 2 to 4 weeks for a colony to be 1 to 2 centimeters in diameter.
2. Many pathogenic fungi are dimorphic, i.e., exhibit two distinct morphological forms. At room temperature on Sabouraud's agar medium, the fungus may grow in a hyphal or mycelial form and produce spores. If the organism is placed on a somewhat richer medium (e.g., brain-heart infusion agar) and cultured at 35–37 C, the organism forms yeast cells. All the hyphae and spores disappear. The yeast cell form is the tissue phase or the in vivo form of the fungus. If a fungus isolated from a patient is dimorphic, this is a good clue that one is dealing with a pathogen. Observe Figure 1–6.

Fig 1–6.—Dimorphism in a fungus. Above, yeast cells as seen growing in a patient or cultured at 35 C. Below, this is the same fungus but cultured at 25 C. Now this fungus is producing septate hyphae and spores.

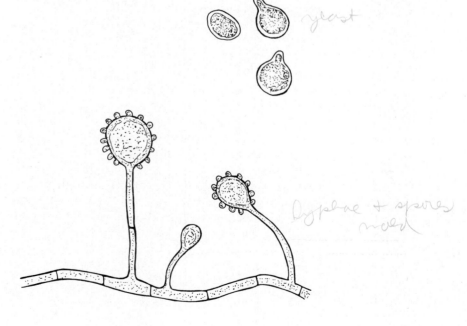

3. The organisms cultured should be examined both grossly and micro-scopically and their morphological features evaluated. Grossly, one should note the texture and color of the colony. Microscopically, one should note whether the hyphae are septate or coenocytic, the manner in which the spores are borne and the size and shape of spores.

4. The most commonly used media for culturing fungi are Sabouraud's agar for room temperature incubation and brain-heart infusion agar for cultur-ing the yeast form of pathogens at 35–37 C. Suspected dermatophytes are cultured at room temperature on Sabouraud's agar and Sabouraud's agar containing cycloheximide and chloramphenicol (e.g., Mycosel or Mycobiotic agar).

SELF-EVALUATION QUESTIONS
(Answers at end of questions)

Check the ONE best answer to each question below:

1. Dematiaceous fungi are
   a. _____ produced in granules
   b. _____ intracellular parasites
   c. _____ brown
   d. _____ coenocytic

2. The medium of choice for culturing the yeast form of dimorphic fungi is
   a. _____ brain-heart infusion
   b. _____ Sabouraud's
   c. _____ Sabouraud's plus antibiotics
   d. _____ any medium incubated at 35–37 C.

3. Which of the following is produced sexually?
   a. _____ ascospore
   b. _____ conidium
   c. _____ oidium
   d. _____ yeast buds

4. Septate and coenocytic are
   a. _____ similar
   b. _____ synonymous
   c. _____ the opposite
   d. _____ forms of yeasts

5. The fungal nucleus
   a. _____ contains true chromosomes
   b. _____ has a nuclear membrane
   c. _____ differs from the bacterial nucleus
   d. _____ all of the above

6. Fungi are classified in the plant kingdom because they
   a. _____ are achlorophyllous
   b. _____ exhibit sexual reproduction
   c. _____ produce spores
   d. _____ have a true cell wall

7. Fungal spores may be produced
   a. _____ singly
   b. _____ in chains

    c. _____ in a sporangium
    d. _____ all of the above
8. A sporangium contains
    a. _____ spherules
    b. _____ sporangiospores
    c. _____ chlamydospores
    d. _____ oidia
9. Most fungi live as
    a. _____ animal parasites
    b. _____ parasites of trees and other vegetation
    c. _____ saprophytes
    d. _____ normal flora in man
10. *Cryptococcus neoformans* differs from other pathogenic fungi because it
    a. _____ has a capsule
    b. _____ is an intracellular parasite
    c. _____ has septate hyphae
    d. _____ reproduces by binary fission

For the following questions, fill in the blanks:

11. The long, slender tubes produced by fungi are known as _____.
12. A dimorphic fungus is one that produces _____ *yeast* _____ when cultured at 35 – 37 C and ____ *mold* ____ *hyphae + spores* when cultured at room temperature.
13. Hyphae which are not septate are ____ *coenocytic or aseptate* ____.
14. The infectious particle for coccidioidomycosis is the ____ *arthrospore* ____.
15. Yeast cells typically reproduce by ____ *budding* ____.
16. Most of the fungi that cause human disease occur naturally in ____ *soil* ____.
17. Potassium hydroxide is used to prepare pus, sputum and other specimens for direct examination purposes because it _____.
18. Granules that contain relatively large hyphae are from cases of _____.
19. The only organisms that produce both yeast cells and hyphae in vivo are
    _____.
20. Ascospores are produced meiotically inside an ____ *ascus* ____.

Answers to Questions 1 to 20.

1. c	11. hyphae
2. a	12. yeast, hyphae
3. a	13. coenocytic
4. c	14. arthrospore
5. d	15. buds (budding)
6. d	16. soil
7. d	17. dissolves tissue debris
8. b	18. eumycotic mycetoma
9. c	19. *Candida* species
10. a	20. ascus

coverslip and examine microscopically, or heat fix the granules and do a gram stain. Inside the crushed granules look for finely branched filaments.

Culture

To culture the organism, place several granules in a sterile test tube. Wash them several times with sterile water. Some workers add penicillin and streptomycin to the water to reduce the number of bacteria. Decant the water and place the granules in a sterile mortar with sand. Add 1 or 2 milliliters of water. Grind the granules with a pestle to break open the hard, outer rind. Culture the ground-up granules at 37 C on trypticase soy agar or the more commonly used brain-heart infusion agar, *under anaerobic or microaerophilic conditions.* In 2 or 3 days, small, white colonies 1–3 millimeters in diameter appear. Some colonies are rough and some are smooth; these are the R and S forms. After 7–10 days, colonies of *A. israelii* become crater-shaped; this is the characteristic "molar-tooth" colony. In culture, when observed microscopically, the organism tends to fragment and assume coccoidal or bacillary forms which may resemble diphtheroids; however, *Actinomyces* species are catalase negative, while most diphtheroids are catalase positive. As is true with all fungi, *Actinomyces israelii* is gram-positive, although it may be better termed gram-variable.

One development that may be important in the future is the recent discovery of other *Actinomyces* species and *Actinomyces*-like organisms which also cause human diseases, e.g., *A. (Bifidobacterium) eriksonii, A. naeslundii* and *Arachnia propionica.* Some of these species have been isolated from diseased lacrimal ducts and lungs.

Other Laboratory Tests

Animal inoculations are not useful in diagnosing actinomycosis. There are no serological tests that are of any diagnostic value. Definitive diagnosis is made by the clinical picture, isolation of granules, culture and microscopic identification of the etiologic agent.

Therapy

Penicillin is the drug of choice. High doses (3–5 million units/day) are administered over a long period, treatment being continued for some time after there is a clinical cure. Streptomycin is used in patients sensitive to penicillin. Sometimes the lesion is treated by radiation and surgical removal or drainage.

Slides

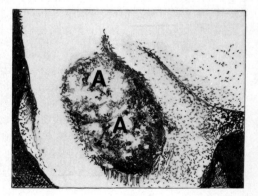

Slide 2–1.—This is the typical lesion (A) seen in actinomycosis. The lesion is in the cervicofacial area and probably took several months to reach this state. If the disease is allowed to progress, draining sinus tracts will develop, and the characteristic sulfur granules will be found in the exudate.

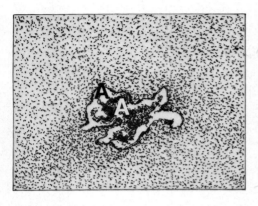

Slide 2–2.—This is typical of a sulfur granule (A) from a case of actinomycosis. The size of these granules is such that they can be seen by the naked eye. One can collect these granules by aspirating a sinus tract. If enough fluid is collected, it should be dispensed into a sterile test tube. By holding this test tube up to the light, one can frequently see the yellow-to-sulfur-colored granules settling out at the bottom of the tube. Another way to collect granules is to place a thick gauze bandage over a sinus tract. The next morning when the bandage is removed, it should be possible to see many of the granules adhering to the gauze.

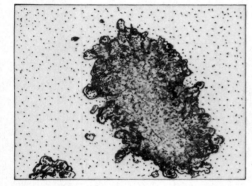

Slide 2–3.—Here is another sulfur granule from a case of actinomycosis. This particular granule was placed on a microscope slide and observed under low magnification.

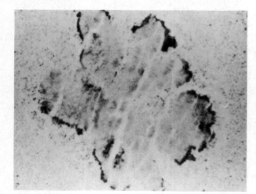

Slide 2–4.—In the middle of this stained tissue section one can see a large granule. Note the lobulated shape of the granule and the ragged outer edges.

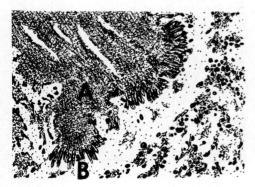

Slide 2–5.—This is a higher magnification of a sulfur granule in tissue. Approximately three fourths of this slide, the darker (red-stained) area (A), is taken up by the granule. The edge of the granule is very ragged (B) and has numerous finger-like clubs projecting out of it.

Slide 2–6. — This is a stained photomicrograph from a culture of *Actinomyces israelii*. The organism shows a definite tendency to form long strands of very fine, delicate filaments which are less than 1 micron in diameter.

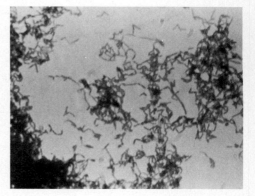

Slide 2–7. — These *A. israelii* colonies were cultured for 8 – 10 days anaerobically on brain-heart infusion agar. They are often referred to as "molar-tooth" colonies.

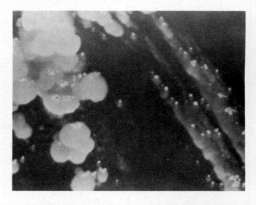

Slide 2–8. — This is the organism growing in a tube of thioglycolate medium. It grows deep in the tube, where less oxygen is available, because *A. israelii* requires microaerophilic to anaerobic conditions for growth.

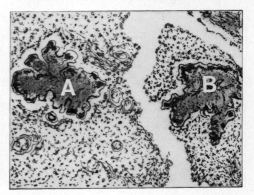

Slide 2–9. — In this slide two granules (A,B) appear to be very similar to the ones previously shown. These are *not* from a case of actinomycosis but are from the disease known as botryomycosis. In stained tissue sections it is nearly impossible to distinguish between actinomycosis and botryomycosis. The latter disease is caused by several other bacteria, and these granules are actually microcolonies of bacteria. This slide shows that the microscopic morphology of granules in tissue is not completely diagnostic for actinomycosis.

NOCARDIOSIS

Synonym

None.

Definition

Nocardiosis is primarily a pulmonary disease. It may metastasize to other body organs, especially the brain. It may be either an acute or a chronic disease.

Etiology

In more than 99% of nocardiosis cases, the etiologic agent is *Nocardia asteroides*. *N. asteroides* is not a true fungus. It is classified in the Actinomycetales and thus is a bacterium.

Epidemiology

The etiologic agent of nocardiosis is found worldwide in soil as a saprophyte and may infect any sex or age group. The disease has a particular predilection for the compromised host. Nocardiosis is found in numerous animals, especially the dog, but the disease is not transmitted from animal to man or from man to man.

Clinical Forms

Nocardiosis is primarily a pulmonary disease but is capable of hematogenous dissemination. When dissemination occurs, the organism shows a predilection for the central nervous system, causing pyogenic lesions in the brain or meninges. There are two principal clinical types of nocardiosis:

1. A very rapid, *acute* form; one of the few "fungus" diseases that progresses rapidly, it is most frequently seen in children. It often mimics pneumonia in symptomatology and rapidity of onset. It is so acute that patients may die one or two days after they have been admitted to a hospital.
2. A *chronic* form is found mainly in the elderly or debilitated. It is often found in patients with tuberculosis. This form may take months or even several years to develop.

Predilections

Although any sex or age group may be infected, the acute form of nocardiosis appears to be more prevalent among younger people, while the chronic form is more common in the elderly and debilitated.

Tissue Form and Histopathology

In tissue, *N. asteroides* is best seen with the tissue gram stain (Brown and Brenn). The organism appears as very fine, delicately branched filaments (less than 1 micron in diameter) scattered throughout the tissue. This organism does *not* form granules in the disease nocardiosis.

Direct Microscopic Examination

Direct microscopic examination is very helpful in arriving at a diagnosis. Sputum is the most commonly examined material, although pus, spinal fluid or biopsy material can be examined if available. *Nocardia asteroides* is gram-positive and partially acid-fast. One way to differentiate *N. asteroides* from *Mycobacterium* species, both of which have filaments that appear similar upon direct microscopic examination, is that mycobacteria are more strongly acid-fast than *N. asteroides* and rarely exhibit branching.

Culture

Nocardia asteroides grows readily on Sabouraud's medium at either room temperature or 37 C; it takes 3 to 5 days for visible growth to appear. The colony is not fluffy but is chalky, leathery, wrinkled and white to orange in color. The colony characteristically emits a musty "old library" smell.

The microscopically delicate filaments (less than 1 micron in diameter) are gram-positive, catalase-positive and partially acid-fast. Just as with *Actinomyces* species, the filaments can be seen in coccoidal or bacillary forms.

Other Laboratory Tests

In nocardiosis neither animal inoculations nor serology are of any diagnostic value.

Therapy

N. asteroides is not usually part of man's normal flora. Whenever it is isolated from a patient, it is indicative of a disease process that should be treated.

The classical drug of choice is high-dose sulfadiazine; however, recent publications indicate better results with a combination of sulfamethoxazole and trimethoprim. Dietary improvement and rest are helpful. Surgical intervention is sometimes indicated.

Slides

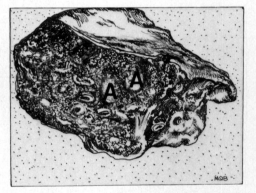

Slide 2–10.—This is lung tissue infected with *Nocardia asteroides* from a fatal human case of pulmonary nocardiosis. Note the numerous slightly colored lesions (A).

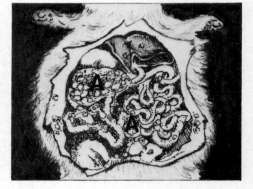

Slide 2–11.—The disease nocardiosis can be readily produced in experimental animals, particularly when the organism is suspended in 5% hog gastric mucin. Note in this guinea pig the numerous light-colored lesions (A) which appear in or on almost every organ.

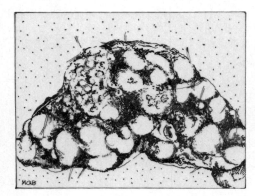

Slide 2–12.—This is tissue removed from the animal shown in Slide 2–11. It is packed solid with very hard, white lesions which contain *Nocardia asteroides.* These lesions are not granules.

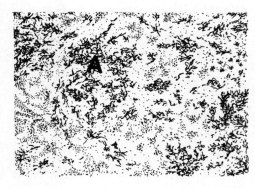

Slide 2–13.—This is a methenamine silver stain (GMS) prepared from a human case of nocardiosis. All of the black color in this slide (A) is the organism *Nocardia asteroides.* This slide was taken under relatively low magnification, which makes it difficult to discern individual filaments.

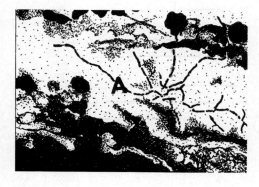

Slide 2–14.—Using the oil immersion lens, one sees the organism *Nocardia asteroides* stained with a modified acid-fast stain (A). Note that the fine filaments (which are pink-stained) in the center of the picture closely resemble an atypical *Mycobacterium* such as *M. fortuitum.*

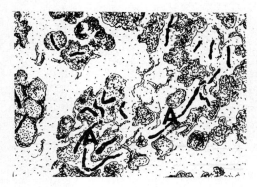

Slide 2–15.—This is a high-magnification photomicrograph of a tissue gram stain preparation of lung infected with *Nocardia asteroides.* The organism (A) can be seen in the center of the slide as very fine, delicate filaments which are less than 1 micron in diameter.

Slide 2–16.—This is another photomicrograph of *Nocardia asteroides* in tissue stained by the gram method, showing that some microorganisms react strangely to gram stain. In the center of this slide (A) are numerous delicate filaments which look blotchy because only certain areas in the filaments are gram-positive.

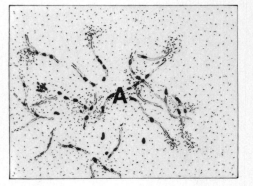

Slide 2–17.—This is the gross appearance of a 4- to 5-week-old culture of *Nocardia asteroides* on Sabouraud's medium. The colony is very compact, hard and rough. For many strains of *Nocardia asteroides,* the vivid orange color is characteristic; however, many isolates do not produce such an intense orange olor and some strains are almost pure white. All of these cultures have a musty, "old library" smell.

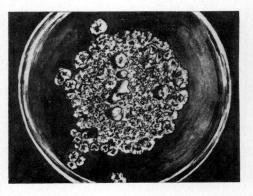

Slide 2–18.—This is the microscopic appearance of *Nocardia asteroides,* prepared from a laboratory culture. There is nothing particularly distinguishing about it except that the organism produces very fine, delicate, branching filaments.

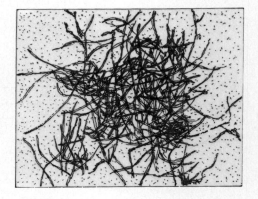

MYCETOMA

Synonyms

Madura foot, maduromycosis.

Definition

Mycetoma is a chronic granulomatous infection, which produces tumor-like lesions and sinus tract formation with the presence of granules, usually of the foot. Skin and subcutaneous tissues are involved originally, but as the disease progresses fascia and bone become infected.

Etiology

More than 15 different organisms are known to cause mycetoma. All of these induce a similar clinical picture and form granules in vivo. The etiologic agents are divided into two distinct groups:

1. *Actinomycotic*. These organisms belong in the Actinomycetales, e.g., *Actinomadura, Nocardia* and *Streptomyces*, species. The granules produced by these organisms contain very fine, delicate filaments (less than 1 micron in diameter).

2. *Eumycotic* (true fungi). These etiologic agents are true filamentous fungi. In eumycotic mycetoma, the granules contain large, coarse, septate hyphae (5–10 microns in diameter). *Allescheria* (or Petriellidium), *Madurella* and *Phialophora* species are most commonly implicated as etiologic agents.

Epidemiology

All of the mycetoma-causing organisms grow in soil as saprophytes. The disease is found worldwide but is most common in Central and South America, Africa and India. In general, mycetoma occurs near or south of the equator. In these areas, it is a very common disease; for example, some African hospitals see up to 3,000 cases a year on an outpatient basis alone.

Clinical Forms

Actinomycotic and eumycotic mycetoma have the same clinical appearance. The foot is the most commonly infected part of the body. As the disease progresses, the foot becomes grossly deformed. Advanced cases have multiple fistulae which drain from the underlying abscesses.

Predilections

As the mycetoma-causing organisms live in the soil, mycetoma is more common among people who have a great deal of contact with the soil. The disease is usually contracted through a puncture wound in the foot.

Tissue Form and Histopathology

Infected tissue may be stained with hematoxylin and eosin (H&E), periodic acid-Schiff (PAS), Brown and Brenn (tissue gram) or methenamine silver (GMS).

Under low-power magnification, the tissue contains numerous, discrete granules. These vary in size, shape, color and morphology, depending on the specific etiologic agent involved. Using higher magnification, one sees true septate hyphae and numerous chlamydospores in the granules of eumycotic mycetoma or very fine filamentous to bacillary or coccoid forms in the granules of actinomycotic mycetoma.

Direct Microscopic Examination

Obtain some pus or other exudate from a draining sinus tract and examine it for granules. By observing the size, color and general morphology of the granules, it is possible to obtain a preliminary indication of what etiologic agent is involved. Place some of the exudate on a microscope slide and add a drop or two of 10–20% KOH. Break open the granules and add a coverslip. If the granules contain septate hyphae and chlamydospores, one is dealing with

eumycotic mycetoma; if they contain fine filaments, it is actinomycotic mycetoma. Additionally, the acid-fast characteristics of the organism help to differentiate among some of the etiologic agents.

Culture

Culturing the organism is not usually necessary for a general diagnosis. If
one decides to confirm and be more specific with the diagnostic suspicion by
culture, the recommended media are Sabouraud's dextrose agar (SDA) and
brain-heart infusion agar (BHI). Antibacterial antibiotics are used rarely in
these media because they may inhibit the aerobic actinomycetes, which cause
actinomycotic mycetoma. Room temperature incubation for 3–6 weeks is
recommended. Each of the organisms has different cultural characteristics; a
description of them can be found in mycology texts.

Other Laboratory Tests

Animal inoculations are of no diagnostic value. Serologic tests are available
but are rarely needed diagnostically.

Therapy

It is very important to differentiate between actinomycotic and eumycotic
mycetoma because the two diseases are treated differently and have different
prognoses. Actinomycotic mycetoma often responds to antibacterial antibiotics of the type used for gram-positive bacterial infections. For eumycotic
mycetoma, there is no effective therapy except amputation of the infected ex-
tremity.

Slides

Slide 2–19.—This picture demonstrates that the disease maduromycosis
can occur in areas other than the foot.
This patient probably has had this disease for several years. Despite the appearance, the patient probably feels very
little pain, and his ability to walk about is
scarcely affected.

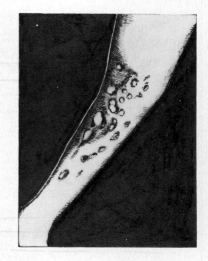

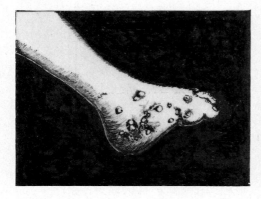

Slide 2–20.—This is a more typical
case of maduromycosis. This patient has
probably had this disease for many years.
Again, he feels very little pain. The disease was probably allowed to develop to
this state because the patient, realizing
that amputation would probably be the
treatment recommended, was reluctant
to go to the hospital.

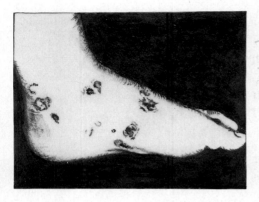

Slide 2–21.—This is another very typical case of madura foot. Note the development of sinus tracts. It is from these tracts that the characteristic granules can be obtained. The size, shape, color and general morphology of these granules are important diagnostically. Additionally, it is from these granules that one cultures the etiologic agent. As with actinomycosis, it is best to wash the granules in an antibiotic solution to eliminate contaminating bacteria. The granules are then ground with sterile sand and cultured on Sabouraud's medium at room temperature.

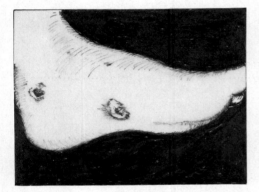

Slide 2–22.—This is the only case of eumycotic mycetoma that we have seen in our medical center. The etiologic agent was *Allescheria boydii*. As far as we can determine, this patient contracted the disease in her back yard from a puncture wound in her foot. At the time this picture was taken, the patient reported that she had had this problem for 4–5 years. To this date, we have been unable to cure her disease.

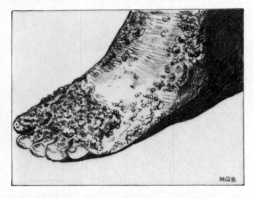

Slide 2–23.—This is a typical case of mycetoma in a patient from South America.

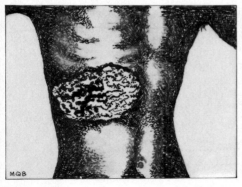

Slide 2–24.—This is an unusual case of mycetoma seen in an African patient.

Slide 2–25.—The dark structure (which is stained red) in this slide is a granule (A) from madura foot. Note that it is very similar to the granules of actinomycosis; of course, the clinical picture is usually quite different.

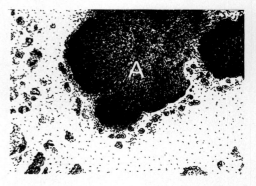

Slide 2–26.—The large structures (A) in the center of this photograph show another type of granule seen in maduromycosis.

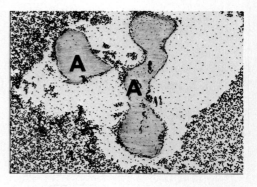

Slide 2–27.—This is another example of a granule (A) in maduromycosis. In this slide, the granule is the huge spherical structure in the middle of the photograph.

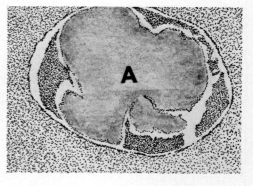

Slide 2–28.—This is another type of granule (A) seen in mycetoma. Note the thick, dark outer rind on this granule.

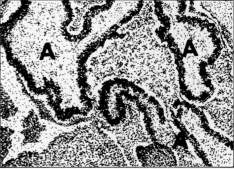

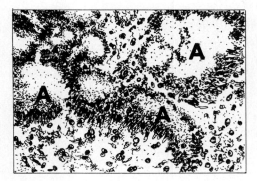

Slide 2–29.—In this slide, there is a granule of actinomycotic mycetoma. The granule is the darker, stained structure which takes up the majority of the slide (A). Close examination of its internal composition shows that it is made up of numerous, very fine, delicate filaments which are less than 1 micron in diameter.

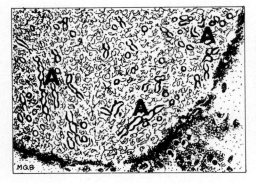

Slide 2–30.—The entire structure in this photomicrograph is a granule from a case of eumycotic mycetoma. Note that inside this granule one can discern numerous relatively large septate hyphae (A). The presence of hyphae of this type inside a granule is diagnostic for eumycotic mycetoma.

The etiologic agents of both types of mycetoma are too numerous to present here. However, the next 2 slides show one of the more common etiologic agents, *Allescheria boydii*, or, as it is referred to in some books, *Monosporium apiospermum*. Recently, taxonomists have agreed that the name *Allescheria boydii* should be changed to *Petriellidium boydii*.

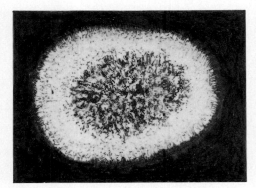

Slide 2–31.—This is a gross culture of the organism *Allescheria boydii* cultured at room temperature on Sabouraud's medium for 3 weeks. This organism is quite fluffy, and the hyphae are white to gray. The underside of this colony is a gray to brown color.

Slide 2–32.—This is a photomicrograph which shows the characteristic spores of *A. boydii*. The spores (A) are the numerous round to pyriform structures scattered along the hyphae. The spores are 5–10 microns in diameter. This organism is one of many true fungi which cause eumycotic mycetoma.

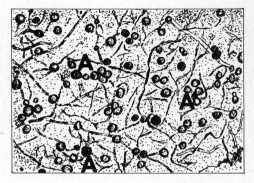

SELF-EVALUATION QUESTIONS
(Answers at end of questions)

Check the ONE best answer to each question below:

1. In vivo, the etiologic agents of the mycetomas are seen
   a. _____ as encapsulated yeast
   b. _____ as septate hyphae
   c. _____ in granules
   d. _____ inside histiocytes

2. Many so-called higher bacteria are classified in the
   a. _____ Actinomycetales
   b. _____ genus *Nocardia*
   c. _____ genus *Streptomyces*
   d. _____ true fungi

3. The most common clinical form of actinomycosis is
   a. _____ cervicofacial
   b. _____ visceral
   c. _____ abdominal
   d. _____ cutaneous

4. In most cases of mycetoma, the sinus tracts yield
   a. _____ large, septate hyphae
   b. _____ yeast cells
   c. _____ coenocytic hyphae
   d. _____ granules

5. Actinomycotic mycetoma differs from eumycotic mycetoma in
   a. _____ clinical characteristics
   b. _____ production of granules
   c. _____ production of sinus tracts
   d. _____ size of the intragranular hyphae

6. In vivo, *Nocardia asteroides* reproduces
   a. _____ as delicate filaments
   b. _____ inside granules
   c. _____ as coenocytic hyphae
   d. _____ in sinus tracts

7. The etiologic agents of mycetomas grow in nature as
   a. _____ soil saprophytes
   b. _____ plant pathogens
   c. _____ animal pathogens
   d. _____ normal flora of man
8. Which of the following organisms is microaerophilic?
   a. _____ *Allescheria* (or *Petriellidium*) *boydii*
   b. _____ *Nocardia asteroides*
   c. _____ *Monosporium apiospermum*
   d. _____ *Actinomyces israelii*
9. Which of the following diseases has numerous etiologic agents?
   a. _____ actinomycosis
   b. _____ nocardiosis
   c. _____ mycetoma
   d. _____ all of the above
10. The endemic area for actinomycosis and nocardiosis is
    a. _____ worldwide
    b. _____ eastern United States
    c. _____ any tropical region
    d. _____ western United States

For the following questions, fill in the blanks.

11. The disease actinomycosis is _____ in origin.
12. Some investigators feel that _____ is a predisposing factor to actinomycosis.
13. In histopathology sections, *Actinomyces israelii* is seen as _____.
14. For cases of actinomycosis, the drug of choice is _____.
15. Nocardiosis is primarily a _____ disease.
16. In tissue, the organism *Nocardia asteroides* is difficult to differentiate from _____.
17. *Nocardia asteroides* grows readily on _____ medium.
18. Maduromycosis is usually contracted through _____.
19. Cases of actinomycotic mycetoma may respond to _____.
20. *Allescheria* (or *Petriellidium*) *boydii* is one of the causes of _____.

Answers to Questions 1 to 20.

1. c	11. endogenous
2. a	12. poor oral hygiene, trauma
3. a	13. sulfur granules
4. d	14. penicillin
5. d	15. pulmonary
6. a	16. *Mycobacterium* species
7. a	17. Sabouraud's
8. d	18. puncture wounds
9. c	19. antibacterial antibiotics
10. a	20. eumycotic mycetoma

3 / Blastomycosis, Paracoccidioidomycosis and Sporotrichosis

BLASTOMYCOSIS

Synonyms

Gilchrist's disease, Chicago disease, North American blastomycosis.

Definition

Blastomycosis is a chronic infection found mainly in lungs. It is characterized by suppurative and granulomatous lesions and is readily confused with other systemic mycoses or neoplasms. If skin lesions develop, they have a characteristic appearance.

Etiology

The only etiologic agent of blastomycosis is *Blastomyces dermatitidis*. The perfect (i.e., sexual) stage is called *Ajellomyces dermatitidis*.

Epidemiology

The major endemic area of the world is the Mississippi River Valley Basin in the United States (Fig 3–1). However, since 1950, cases have been reported in other parts of the world, notably North Africa. Perhaps further investigation will reveal that blastomycosis is worldwide. The organism is thought to grow in soil; however, it has rarely been cultured from nature.

Clinical Forms

There are three principal clinical forms of blastomycosis.
1. *Pulmonary*. The fungus enters the human body via the lung. The infected individual initially has mild respiratory symptoms, such as fever, cough and hoarseness. After a few months, the infection progresses, and the patient then has productive cough, fever and eventually weight loss. Radiographically, the disease looks like tuberculosis, carcinoma or some other chronic respiratory problems.
2. *Systemic*. The systemic form of blastomycosis is an extension of the pulmonary form. The most common sites of involvement are liver and spleen. Granulomatous lesions are present, and abscesses often occur.
3. *Cutaneous*. Most mycologists believe that the presence of cutaneous lesions indicates systemic disease, although some still think that skin lesions may result from direct inoculation from the soil.

The cutaneous lesions of blastomycosis are very characteristic. Lesions develop slowly and after months or years cover large areas of the skin, several inches in diameter. The lesions appear crusty, are elevated 1–3 millimeters and have well-defined margins, which often contain small microabscesses.

Predilections

The ages of reported cases range from 6 to 80 years. However, in one study of 347 cases, 50% of the patients were between 20 and 40 years of age. Nine

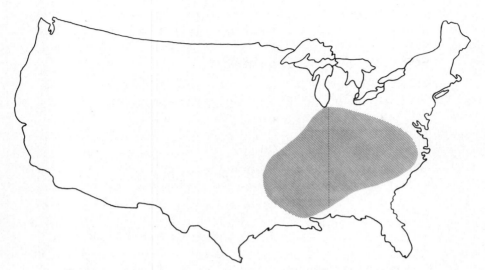

Fig 3–1. – Endemic area for blastomycosis in the United States.

times as many men as women contract blastomycosis. There is no proved occupational predilection, but most persons with the disease seem to have more than normal contact with the soil.

Tissue Form and Histopathology

Blastomyces dermatitidis grows as a yeast in tissue. The yeast cell is thick-walled and 8–15 microns in diameter. Not all of the yeast cells will be budding, but, in those that are, look for an enlarged point of attachment where the bud meets the parent cell; this is the "broad-based bud." *Blastomyces dermatitidis* is the only yeast that characteristically reproduces in animals with a broad-based bud.

Direct Microscopic Examination

In the pulmonary form, sputum is useful for diagnosis; with cutaneous lesions, skin scrapings from the periphery of the lesions are best. Biopsy material can also be used. Place the material on a microscope slide in 1–2 drops of 10–20% KOH (to clear out cellular debris) and look for broad-based yeast cells. This is a quick and simple test and should be done whenever blastomycosis is suspected.

Culture

Blastomycoses dermatitidis is a true dimorphic fungus. At room temperature (on Sabouraud's, Mycosel or Mycobiotic agar) it grows into a fluffy, white to brownish-white fungus which produces small aleuriospores (5 microns) after 2–3 weeks' incubation. The aleuriospores are thought to be the infectious particles. If the hyphae from the room temperature culture are incubated on brain-heart infusion agar at 37 C, after 2–3 weeks yeast cells identical to those seen in vivo are formed.

Other Laboratory Tests

Animal inoculation works well but is impractical to do routinely. There is a skin test material available called "blastomycin," but in my opinion, it is of little value because of its cross-reactivity with many other diseases. At best, a positive response to blastomycin means that the patient may have a fungus disease. Some serologic tests are available, but the interpretation of results is controversial.

Therapy

Amphotericin B is the drug of choice but is only erratically successful. Certain cases respond to therapy with 2-hydroxystilbamidine.

Slides

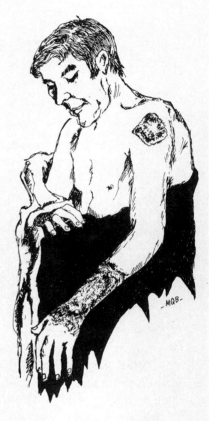

Slide 3–1.—This is one of the more typical clinical pictures of blastomycosis. In this particular case, the skin lesions are manifestations of internal disease. Note the lesion on the left shoulder and the larger one on the left wrist.

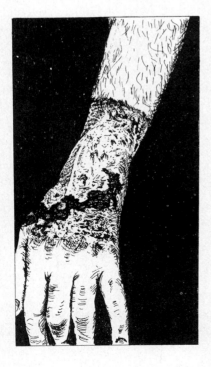

Slide 3–2.—This is a close-up of the wrist lesion shown in Slide 3–1. Note the well-defined margin of the lesion.

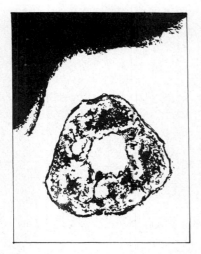

Slide 3–3.—This is the lesion seen on the shoulder of the patient in Slide 3–1. Note that this lesion is very rough, somewhat elevated and very precisely marginated. It is characteristic of blastomycosis, and many clinicians consider it highly diagnostic for this disease. When one wishes to remove material from this lesion for culture or direct examination procedures, it is best to select material near the edge of the lesion. It is a characteristic of fungus diseases that the outer portion of a lesion is the area in which the fungus is most actively growing.

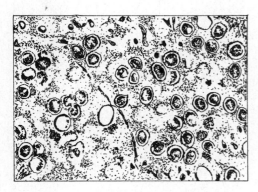

Slide 3–4.—This is a tissue section from a case of blastomycosis. The slide is filled with yeast cells that are 10–12 microns in diameter. Some of these yeast cells appear to have a thin, clear halo around them. This is the thick cell wall of the fungus.

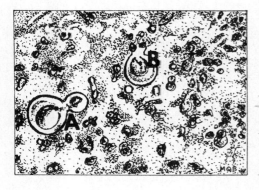

Slide 3–5.—This is a higher magnification photomicrograph showing two yeast cells of *Blastomyces dermatitidis* (A,B) growing in human tissue. In this particular picture, the cytoplasm inside the yeast cells has contracted, giving the erroneous appearance that the organism has a capsule. This contraction of the protoplasm is a fixation artifact. Most important, note that one of the yeast cells has a bud on it (A). At the point where the bud is attached to the parent yeast cell the area is quite thick and spread out; this is known as a broad-based bud, which is diagnostic for the organism *Blastomyces dermatitidis.*

Slide 3–6.—This is what one would expect to see by examining skin scrapings, sputum or biopsy material using the direct examination method, namely, placing the material on a microscope slide with 1–2 drops of 10–20% KOH. (For photographic purposes some blue dye was added.) Three or four spherical yeast cells are 8–15 microns in diameter. One of these yeast cells, off to the side of the photograph (A), is in the process of budding. Note the characteristic broad-based bud.

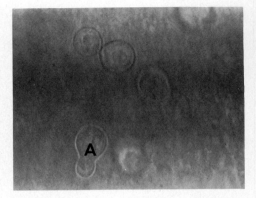

Slide 3–7.—This is a culture of *Blastomyces dermatitidis* grown on Sabouraud's agar at room temperature for 3–4 weeks. This organism usually grows as a completely white, fluffy fungus. The underside of the colony may be a slightly tan to brown color, and some isolates appear to have a slightly reddish color on the underside of the colony.

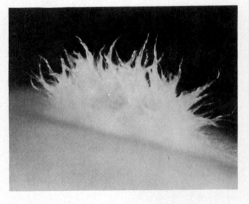

Slide 3–8.—This is a relatively young culture of *B. dermatitidis,* incubated in a test tube for 7 days on Sabouraud's agar medium at room temperature. Note the tufts of aerial hyphae; these projections are referred to as coremia. Many strains of this organism produce coremia in the early stages of growth when cultured in this way.

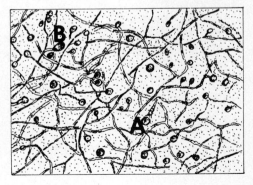

Slide 3–9.—This is a high-power microscopic view of the organism as it grows at room temperature. There are numerous, very delicate, septate hyphae. The small, spherical to pyriform structures are the aleuriospores (A,B). We suspect that these are the infectious particles for blastomycosis. The spores are approximately 5 microns in diameter. This may be the way the organism grows in soil.

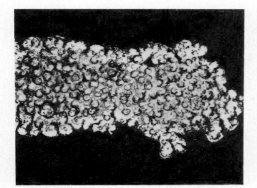

Slide 3–10.—This is the same organism that was observed growing in Slides 3–7 and 3–8, except that it has been cultured on brain-heart infusion agar at 35 to 37 C. This particular colony is probably 3–5 weeks old. Note that this culture is radically different from the room temperature culture; at room temperature there is a completely white, fluffy mold, but at 35 C there is a very rough, dry-appearing yeast colony. This is what is meant by the term "dimorphic fungus."

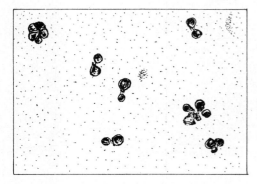

Slide 3–11.—This is a microscopic view of the yeast phase of *Blastomyces dermatitidis*. This preparation was made from the culture seen in Slide 3–10. The yeast cells in this slide are approximately 10–12 microns in diameter and reproduce by forming broad-based buds.

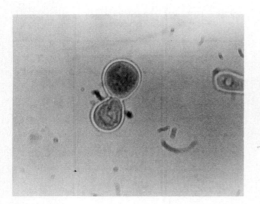

Slide 3–12.—This is a higher magnification of a yeast cell like those seen in Slide 3–11. Again the mode of attachment of the new bud to the parent yeast cell, namely, the formation of a broad-based bud, is apparent.

PARACOCCIDIOIDOMYCOSIS

Synonyms

South American blastomycosis, "para" or "paracocci."

Definition

Paracoccidioidomycosis is a chronic granulomatous disease of skin, mucous membranes, lymph nodes and internal organs.

Etiology

The etiologic agent of paracoccidioidomycosis is *Paracoccidioides brasiliensis*. The yeast cells of *Paracoccidioides brasiliensis* are larger than those of *Blastomyces dermatitidis* and have multiple small buds.

Epidemiology

This disease is very common in South America, especially in Brazil. Outside South America it is seldom seen. The organism probably resides in soil.

Clinical Forms

Paracoccidioidomycosis most commonly involves nasal and oral mucosa, with resulting enlargement of lymph nodes. Cutaneous lesions often develop on the face. In rare instances, dissemination to a variety of internal organs may occur.

Predilections

Nine times as many men as women contract paracoccidioidomycosis. This is probably because of greater contact with the soil. The predominant, but by no means exclusive, age group is between 20 and 30 years. Like *Blastomyces dermatitidis*, *Paracoccidioides brasiliensis* is thought to live in soil, but this has not been proved.

Tissue Form and Histopathology

In tissue, *Paracoccidioides brasiliensis* produces large yeast cells that are about 10–30 microns in diameter. The yeast cells have numerous small buds on them, giving the overall appearance of a mariner's wheel.

Direct Microscopic Examination

This is easier and quicker than sectioning fixed tissue. Place some material on a microscope slide and add 1–2 drops of 10–20% KOH and a coverslip. Press down on the coverslip to spread out the tissue. Examine microscopically for the presence of large (10–30 microns) yeast cells which have multiple buds (1–2 microns in diameter).

Culture

Paracoccidioides brasiliensis is a dimorphic pathogen. At room temperature on Sabouraud's agar it grows as a non-spore-forming, septate fungus; on brain-heart infusion agar at 37 C it produces the yeast form that is seen in tissue.

Other Laboratory Tests

Some serologic tests are available and are highly reliable. Complement fixation and immunodiffusion tests are the most widely used.

Therapy

For paracoccidioidomycosis, amphotericin B is the drug of choice.

Slides

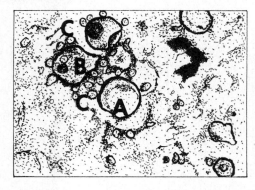

Slide 3–13. — Here one sees the development of a chronic granulomatous disease in which the lymph nodes of the neck are involved. In other cases, skin or mucous membranes and, rarely, internal organs are infected. This is a case of paracoccidioidomycosis.

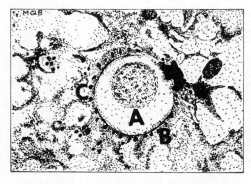

Slide 3–14. — This is how the etiologic agent, *Paracoccidioides brasiliensis,* grows in tissue. In this slide are several rather large yeast cells (A,B), which are usually 10–30 microns in diameter. Many very small (1 micron in diameter) buds project out of some of the yeast cells (C).

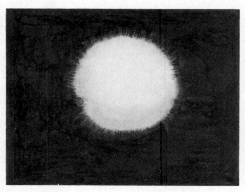

Slide 3–15. — In the center of this field is a large yeast cell of *Paracoccidioides brasiliensis* (A). In this particular photograph, the cytoplasm has shrunk into the middle of the cell, giving the erroneous impression that the organism is encapsulated. The important part of this picture is that this yeast cell is surrounded by at least two dozen darkly stained, very minute buds (B,C): this is known as multiple budding.

Slide 3–16. — This is a culture of *Paracoccidioides brasiliensis* grown on Sabouraud's agar at room temperature for 3–4 weeks. This colony is very fluffy and is composed of pure white hyphae. Microscopically, the hyphae are sterile, which means that they lack spores.

Slide 3–17.—This is the same organism seen in Slide 3–16, except that it has been cultured at 35–37 C on brain-heart infusion agar for 3–5 weeks. This fungus is dimorphic, which means that at 35 C it does not form filamentous hyphae but, instead, produces a pure yeast colony. Microscopically, the yeast cells from this culture are 10–30 microns in diameter and contain numerous (15–30) very minute (1–2 microns in diameter) buds.

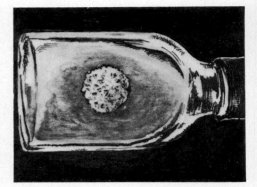

Slide 3–18.—This slide and Slide 3–19 show a disease referred to as Lobo's disease. This disease is restricted to natives who have lived for extended periods of time in the Amazon area of Brazil. Many persons consider Lobo's disease an unusual clinical form of paracoccidioidomycosis. Much confusion still exists over this disease because, to this date, the etiologic agent has not been cultured from nature or from clinical cases.

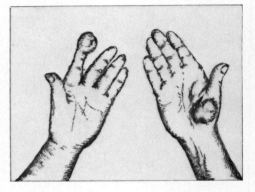

Slide 3–19.—This is a more advanced form of Lobo's disease. The patient has undoubtedly had this disease for many years. Despite the rather verrucous nature of these lesions, the patient has little pain and is still able to walk with only minor difficulty. (Slide courtesy of J. W. Rippon, from *Medical Mycology,* 1974.)

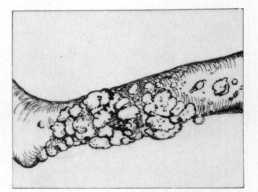

SPOROTRICHOSIS

Synonym

Gardener's disease.

Definition

Sporotrichosis is a chronic, subcutaneous mycosis with eventual lymphatic involvement. In some advanced, untreated cases, it may become a generalized infection and involve bones, joints and other internal organs.

Etiology

The etiologic agent of sporotrichosis is *Sporothrix schenckii,* a true dimorphic fungus. It is a common inhabitant of soil and the epidermis of many plants. The avenue of infection is often a scratch from a rose bush (or other thorny plants), forcing the fungus into the subcutaneous tissues.

Epidemiology

Sporotrichosis occurs worldwide and is a relatively common disease.

Clinical Forms

Sporotrichosis is the only fungus disease that can almost always be diagnosed from its clinical picture alone. The typical history and clinical appearance are as follows: The patient receives a scratch from a bush. At first, he has a small, movable, subcutaneous nodule; in about a week's time, the nodule becomes fixed. Later, other nodules appear, and eventually lesions spread up the lymph channels of the arm. Usually there is little pain or malaise associated with the primary stages of sporotrichosis. Occasionally, the lesions become granulomatous and drain. Often, open lesions become secondarily infected with bacteria.

Predilections

Although anyone who comes in contact with the organism can be infected, sporotrichosis shows a distinct predilection for horticultural workers, both professional and amateur. Several years ago, there was a massive outbreak of sporotrichosis among miners in South Africa, owing to contact with mine timbers laden with *Sporothrix schenckii.*

Tissue Form and Histopathology

For practical purposes, *Sporothrix schenckii* is usually not seen in human tissue.

Direct Microscopic Examination

This is rarely helpful.

Culture

Besides the characteristic clinical picture, culture is the only effective way to diagnose sporotrichosis. At room temperature, on Sabouraud's medium (or Mycosel or Mycobiotic), the organism grows out in about 5–10 days. The colony is brown to black, with a greasy-looking appearance. Microscopically, one sees very fine, septate hyphae and aleuriospores, which grow in daisy-like (rosette) clusters. The aleuriospores are the infectious particles.

At 35–37 C on brain-heart infusion agar, the colony changes to a tan-colored yeast. These yeast cells are elongated (8–10 microns long) and gram stain black. Because of their shape and gram stain reaction, the yeast cells of *Sporothrix schenckii* are called cigar bodies.

Other Laboratory Tests

No other laboratory tests are needed for diagnosis of the lymphatic form. Serologic tests are available as aids in diagnosing disseminated sporotrichosis.

Therapy

In the primary stages, before systemic involvement, sporotrichosis is easily and cheaply treated with potassium iodide taken orally. When there is systemic involvement, potassium iodide seldom works. Amphotericin B has been tried for systemic sporotrichosis but has met with little or no success.

Slides

Slide 3–20.—This is the characteristic clinical picture seen in more than 90% of the cases of sporotrichosis. Usually the patient is a horticultural worker or a weekend gardener. The patient may recall pruning his rosebushes or cutting down some thorny bushes several months previously, at which time he received a small scratch on his hand or one of his fingers. After a period of several days, he may recall that a small, subcutaneous nodule began to develop. At first, this nodule was quite movable, but after a week or so it began to adhere to the tissue. At this point, he may have gone to see a physician, who suggested that it was either bacterial in origin or caused by a spider bite. After the usual round of antibiotics, the lesion persisted and, in fact, another one began to appear. At this point, the lesion began to turn purple. Over the next several weeks or months, the lesions began to spread up the lymph channels of the arm, as seen in this particular clinical picture. Note the very distinct cording effect. At this point, one should begin to suspect sporotrichosis and, in fact, the leading question at this time might be, "How do you feel?" If the patient replies that he is feeling fine, then sporotrichosis is a possible diagnosis. As the lesions extend farther up the arm, always following the lymph channels, an occasional lesion may suppurate and drain. Some of these lesions may be secondarily invaded with bacteria.

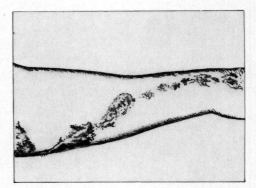

Slide 3–21.—This is another typical case of sporotrichosis. Note the cording effect and that the organism follows the lymph channels up the arm (ascending lymphangitis). This type of clinical picture should immediately call to mind the fungus disease sporotrichosis.

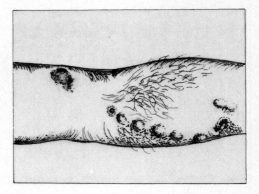

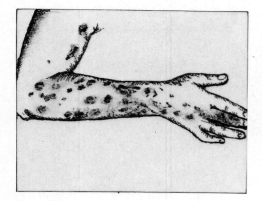

Slide 3–22.—This is a more advanced case of sporotrichosis. The patient has probably had this disease for several months. The distinct cording is more difficult to see in this case, and there is more inflammation present, probably because of a secondary invasion by bacteria.

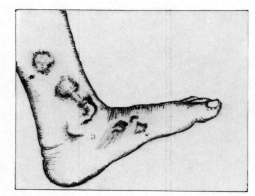

Slide 3–23.—This is a case of sporotrichosis of the foot and leg. We rarely see this form in the United States because most persons here wear shoes. However, in other parts of the world where footwear is not so commonly worn, it is not unusual to see this form of sporotrichosis. This particular case was seen in the central highlands of Vietnam. The patient worked in a horticultural area of that country.

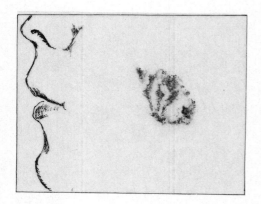

Slide 3–24.—This form of sporotrichosis is deceptive. Occasionally, one sees solitary lesions developing on the neck and face, as in this case. Because the characteristic cording effect is not seen, this form of the disease frequently defies diagnosis. A few years ago at our medical center, we saw numerous cases of this type of sporotrichosis. We were able to determine that all of the infected children had been on a hayride 2 or 3 months previously. During the hayride, all of the participants had a jolly time stuffing hay down one another's necks. Upon examination, we found that the fungus was growing on this hay and that the children had spent the evening inoculating one another with the fungus.

Slide 3–25.—This is another example of the solitary lesion type of sporotrichosis. These lesions have no characteristic features, and direct examination of material is useless. The only way to diagnose this as sporotrichosis is to culture out *Sporothrix schenckii;* fortunately this is not too difficult using Mycosel (or Mycobiotic) agar medium incubated at room temperature.

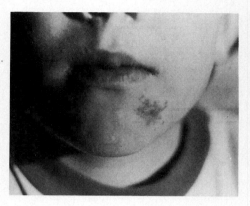

Slide 3–26.—By using gram stain, we see the organism in this smear from the peritoneal cavity of an infected mouse. It is nearly impossible to see this organism in human tissue; however, the organism can be visualized in mouse tissue. In this smear, the organism appears as round (A) to long, slender (B), gram-positive yeast cells which are scattered throughout the entire field. This is probably the way the organism grows in human tissue. Some workers maintain that they are able to see the organism in human tissue when they use a specially devised periodic acid-Schiff stain. However, such specialized stains are not routinely used in clinical laboratories.

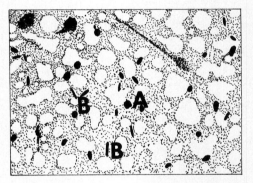

Slide 3–27.—This organism is quite easy to culture in the laboratory. This is a plate of Mycosel agar. *Sporothrix schenckii* colonies completely cover this plate: they are the dark colonies which are surrounded by a white ring. The dark color in these colonies represents the spores; the white ring is the mycelium, which is still too young to produce the darkly colored spores.

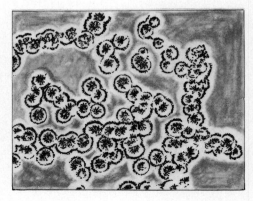

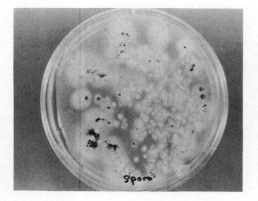

Slide 3–28.—This is the *typical* room temperature culture of *S. schenckii;* however, some isolates (as seen in this picture) remain an off-white color. This lack of coloration is more commonly seen in cultures that have been transferred several times in the laboratory.

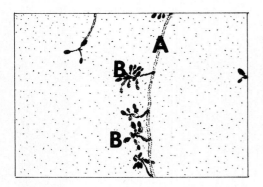

Slide 3–29.—This is a microscopic view of the fungus as it grows at room temperature. This fungus produces extremely fine and delicate hyphae, approximately 3 microns in diameter (A). On the hyphae, the very small aleuriospores (B) are being formed in a floral arrangement. This type of spore arrangement is frequently referred to as a daisy or rosette formation.

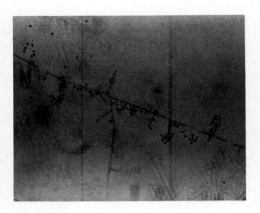

Slide 3–30.—This is another photomicrograph of *S. schenckii* cultured at room temperature. Again note the daisy-like clusters of spores. Also note that the spores in this isolate are not quite as ovate as the spores in Slide 3–29; also some of the spores are produced directly on the hyphae, i.e., not in daisy clusters.

Slide 3–31.—*Sporothrix schenckii* is another dimorphic fungus. This is a gram stain of the organism growing at 35 on brain-heart infusion agar. The entire slide is filled with spherical to long, slender, gram-positive yeast cells. This, we suspect, is the way the organism grows in vivo. As with other dimorphic fungi, if some of these yeast cells were inoculated onto Sabouraud's agar and incubated at room temperature, the result would be the appearance of the filamentous form of this fungus. No more yeast cells would be seen; in their place would be the fine, delicate hyphae and the spores whose arrangement has been described as a daisy cluster or rosette formation. The ability to revert back and forth between the hyphal and yeast forms is the outstanding feature of all dimorphic fungi.

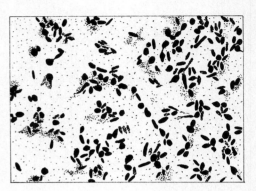

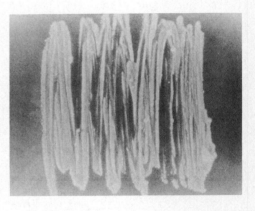

Slide 3–32.—This is *S. schenckii* incubated for 1–2 weeks on brain-heart infusion agar medium at 35–37 C; this is the yeast form. Note how bacteria-like the colonies appear. An off-white to tan color is typical.

SELF-EVALUATION QUESTIONS
(Answers at end of questions)

Check the ONE best answer to each question:

1. The major endemic area for blastomycosis is
   a. _____ Africa
   b. _____ a tropical area
   c. _____ South America
   d. _____ eastern United States
2. *Blastomyces dermatitidis* is thought to reside in nature
   a. _____ in insects
   b. _____ as normal flora of man
   c. _____ in soil
   d. _____ in streams and lakes

3. The important diagnostic feature of *B. dermatitidis* in vivo is
   a. _____ coenocytic hyphae
   b. _____ hyphae less than 1 micron in diameter
   c. _____ granule formation
   d. _____ broad-based yeast cells
4. The skin test material blastomycin is
   a. _____ an important diagnostic tool
   b. _____ used in serologic tests
   c. _____ of prognostic value
   d. _____ of little diagnostic value
5. Growing at room temperature on Sabouraud's medium, *Blastomyces dermatitidis* produces
   a. _____ spherical to pyriform aleuriospores
   b. _____ septate hyphae and no spores
   c. _____ daisy clusters of spores
   d. _____ yeast cells
6. Which one of the following best describes the way *Paracoccidioides brasiliensis* reproduces in vivo?
   a. _____ large yeast cells with many buds
   b. _____ broad-based yeast cells
   c. _____ long, slender yeast cells
   d. _____ pyriform aleuriospores
7. Lobo's disease is probably another form of
   a. _____ mycetoma
   b. _____ blastomycosis
   c. _____ nocardiosis
   d. _____ paracoccidioidomycosis
8. In nature, *Sporothrix schenckii* grows
   a. _____ in water
   b. _____ on domestic animals
   c. _____ on plants and in soil
   d. _____ in soil containing bird excreta
9. "Cigar bodies" refers to
   a. _____ granules seen in mycetoma
   b. _____ any yeast cell
   c. _____ the hyphal form of *Sporothrix schenckii*
   d. _____ the yeast phase of *Sporothrix schenckii*
10. The easiest (and cheapest) mycosis to cure is
    a. _____ pulmonary nocardiosis
    b. _____ sporotrichosis
    c. _____ eumycotic mycetoma
    d. _____ thoracic actinomycosis

For the following questions, fill in the blanks:

11. Most mycologists believe that the presence of cutaneous lesions in blastomycosis indicates _____ disease.
12. *Blastomyces dermatitidis* grows as a _____ in tissue.
13. Because *Blastomyces dermatitidis* produces both yeast and hyphal forms in the laboratory, it is called a _____ fungus.

14. The infectious particle of *Blastomyces dermatitidis* is probably the _____.

15. The drug of choice for blastomycosis is _____.

16. The etiologic agent of paracoccidioidomycosis is _____.

17. Sporotrichosis is most often seen in people who work with _____.

18. Several years ago a large outbreak of sporotrichosis occurred among _____ in South Africa.

19. The yeast phase of *Sporothrix schenckii* is grown on _____ (medium) at _____ (temperature).

20. The drug of choice, for most cases of sporotrichosis, is _____ given _____ (route).

Answers to questions 1 to 20.

1. d	11. systemic
2. c	12. yeast
3. d	13. dimorphic
4. d	14. aleuriospore
5. a	15. amphotericin B
6. a	16. *Paracoccidioides brasiliensis*
7. d	17. plants
8. c	18. miners
9. d	19. brain-heart infusion, 35–37 C
10. b	20. potassium iodide, orally

4 / Coccidioidomycosis and Histoplasmosis

MORE IS KNOWN about coccidioidomycosis and histoplasmosis than any of the other fungus diseases, probably because they both have very large, well-defined endemic areas in North America and are extremely common diseases in the United States. Approximately 50–60 million persons in the United States have been infected with one of these diseases.

Both of these diseases cause acute or chronic lung disease. The chronic form of either disease may readily be mistaken for tuberculosis, various types of cancer and many of the other systemic mycoses.

The organisms which cause these diseases reside in soil and are considered highly infectious. In both instances the inhalation of a single spore usually results in a skin test conversion. *In the laboratory, the room temperature cultures are highly infectious and are a hazard to laboratory personnel.*

COCCIDIOIDOMYCOSIS

Synonyms

"Cocci," desert fever, valley fever, desert rheumatism, "the bumps," San Joaquin Valley fever.

Definition and Clinical Forms

Depending on the author, coccidioidomycosis may be divided into several clinical entities. I have chosen to describe this disease in three clinical forms:

PRIMARY PULMONARY. — This form of the disease occurs 7–28 days after the inhalation of a single spore of the infectious agent. The hallmark of this clinical form is the conversion to a positive skin test. Approximately 80–90% of the persons in the endemic area have or have had this form of the disease. Generally, the symptoms are flu-like, i.e., fever, malaise and cough. Approximately 10% of the infected individuals develop a rash, the so-called erythema nodosum or erythema multiforme. (Immunologically, the development of such rashes is a good sign.) If the disease progresses no further, the individual develops a resistance that may last from 20 years to a lifetime. Serologically, the only important indication of this form is the skin test conversion.

BENIGN FORM. — In cases of this type of coccidioidomycosis not only does the individual become skin test positive but precipitin and complement fixation titers also appear. The hallmark of this form is the development of well-defined lung cavitation, commonly seen as single lesions which may eventually evolve into larger lesions having a diameter of several centimeters. This form of coccidioidomycosis may exist for years; it may go unnoticed, causing the patient no problems, or it may progress into the third form of coccidioidomycosis.

DISSEMINATED FORM. — Fortunately, very few individuals develop disseminated coccidioidomycosis; in fact, fewer than 1 in 200 patients progress to this state. In the disseminated form, coccidioidomycosis spreads into various internal organs, which may include the brain (e.g., meningitis). The prognosis for advanced disseminated cases is grave. Usually in such cases the precipitin titer disappears, the complement fixation titer continues to rise, and a state of anergy (reversion from skin test positive to skin test negative) may exist.

Etiology

The disease coccidioidomycosis is caused by a single organism, *Coccidioides immitis*.

Epidemiology

The major endemic area in the world for coccidioidomycosis is the southwestern part of the United States. Technically, this area is known as a Lower Sonoran Life Zone or the Great Desert Area of the southwestern United States and Mexico. In addition to this endemic area, smaller ones have been found in Central and South America. The possibility still exists that there are other endemic areas in the world.

A Lower Sonoran Life Zone is characterized by little rainfall, extremely high summer temperatures, little vegetation other than cacti and few inhabitants other than rattlesnakes and lizards.

Figure 4–1 shows that the U.S. endemic area includes southern California, Arizona, New Mexico and southwestern Texas. It also extends into Mexico.

In Central and South America, endemic areas are found in Guatemala, Honduras, Venezuela, Paraguay, Argentina and Colombia.

In endemic areas the organism *Coccidioides immitis* resides near the surface of the soil. During the spring, when the desert receives extensive rainfall, the organism flourishes. In this stage, it develops rapidly throughout the soil in a purely mycelial state. When the rains stop and the hot summer begins, the organism grows much more slowly, and the mycelium converts into more re-

Fig 4–1. — Endemic area for coccidioidomycosis in the United States (> 30% population are skin test positive).

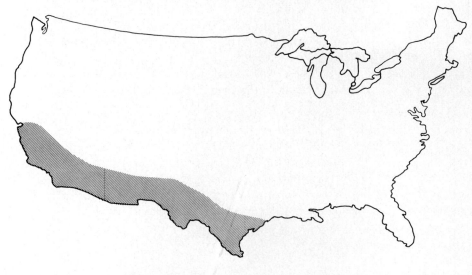

sistant structures, known as arthrospores (arthroaleuriospores). Arthrospores result from hyphal cells. Every other cell seems to increase in size, a thicker wall develops and the cytoplasm appears to "ball up." Such spores can readily break apart from the mycelium and become airborne. In this state, they are approximately 4 by 6 microns and are highly infectious.

Although coccidioidomycosis is commonly found in rodents, snakes and cattle, man never contracts it from any of them. As far as is known, one can only contract this disease by inhalation of arthrospores, and such spores are formed only in the soil or when the organism is grown in the laboratory. Thus *Coccidioides immitis*, when grown in the laboratory, is an extremely dangerous organism. (Note: There are a few reports in the literature of fomite transmission.)

Predilections

A major predisposing factor is actually being in or passing through an endemic area. Aside from this, exposure to excessively large numbers of infectious particles encourages the development of the more serious forms of this disease. Individuals who work with the soil in endemic areas are more susceptible. For some unknown reason it appears that individuals with darker skins are more susceptible than individuals with lighter skins to the disseminated form of coccidioidomycosis. Undoubtedly other factors predispose an individual to the development of the benign or disseminated form, but these are still unknown.

Tissue Form and Histopathology

Although the organism *Coccidioides immitis* may be observed in tissue stained with H&E, the organism is best seen when stained with the PAS method.

Shortly after the arthrospores enter the human body, they convert into a completely different form; thus this organism is dimorphic. In vivo, *Coccidioides immitis* forms thick-walled structures which are known as sporangia or spherules. At first, the sporangia are only 5–10 microns in diameter; however, they soon increase in size. Eventually they reach a diameter of 20–80 microns. Inside these structures numerous spores develop. Such spores are called sporangiospores or endospores. These spores are approximately 5 microns in diameter. As the sporangia or spherules mature and become full of spores, they break open, releasing the spores into the surrounding tissues. These spores then have the capability of developing into sporangia or spherules. Thus, in tissue, *Coccidioides immitis* exhibits considerable variation in size—in fact, much more variation in size than is seen with almost any other fungal pathogen. This variation ranges from the 5 micron endospores up to 80 micron spherules. This is the major way that coccidioidomycosis appears in tissue. In extremely rare instances, hyphal elements are seen, but under no circumstances are yeast cells observed.

Direct Microscopic Examination

Microscopic examination can be most helpful in diagnosing coccidioidomycosis when infected sputum, tissue or skin is available. Place some of this material onto a microscope slide, add 1–2 drops of 10–20% KOH, add a coverslip, heat gently and then press down firmly on the coverslip. Examine this preparation, using the high dry microscope lens. Look for spherules containing endospores. Aside from serologic information, this procedure may afford the first indication that the patient has this mycosis.

Culture

Coccidioides immitis may be cultured rather readily from any infected material, using Sabouraud's medium incubated at room temperature. Under these conditions a fluffy, white fungus develops in 1–3 weeks. The surface of the culture is usually white; however, on the underside there may be some dark brown to gray color seen in the colony. Some isolates appear light pink. In this stage, *Coccidioides immitis* produces arthrospores and thus is an extremely dangerous culture to work with. For reasons of safety, the physician should always inform laboratory personnel that they may be culturing this fungus. They should never try to grow this organism in a Petri dish but should always use test tubes. To make preparations of this culture for a microscopic observation of the hyphae, one should be extremely careful and always work under a hood. Wet the culture and a small portion of the mycelium, place it onto a microscope slide with one or two drops of lactophenol cotton blue, mascerate the mycelium, add a coverslip and observe microscopically, using the high-power lens. At first one observes only masses of rather fine septate hyphae. However, if the culture is *Coccidioides immitis,* one notices that some of the mycelium contains the infectious arthrospores. These cells are usually thicker than regular hyphae, are formed in alternate cells, are approximately 4 by 6 microns, appear to have a thicker wall and are darker blue than the remainder of the hyphal cells. The vast majority of cultures of *Coccidioides immitis* produce arthrospores when grown under the prescribed conditions.

Coccidioides immitis also grows in a mycelial state on Sabouraud's agar, when incubated at 35–37 C; however, at this temperature, the growth may be extremely slow and sparse. In recent years it has been possible, using tissue culture media and conditions, to produce the spherules and endospores in vitro. Since this procedure is rather complicated and of little diagnostic value, it is not done routinely.

Because *Coccidioides immitis* is not inhibited by cycloheximide or any of the antibacterial antibiotics, one may incorporate such materials into the Sabouraud's medium to inhibit overgrowth by various contaminating fungi and bacteria (e.g., Mycosel or Mycobiotic agar).

Other Laboratory Tests

Figure 4–2 is a summary of the serologic picture; such information is important diagnostically, prognostically and therapeutically.

Soon after exposure to the infectious particle, the person becomes skin test positive. The conversion back to skin test negative (anergy) is an indication of a grave prognosis. A precipitin titer develops 1–3 weeks after exposure to the infectious particle. After approximately 2 months, the precipitin titer returns to zero. A positive precipitin titer indicates only that one has had recent contact with this fungus; prognostically and therapeutically, positive precipitin titers are of no value. Approximately 2–3 months after exposure to the infectious particle, the complement fixation titer begins to appear. If this titer continues to rise over extended periods of time, the prognosis is grave. However,

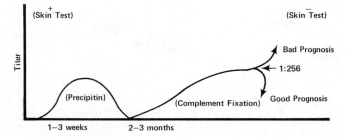

Fig 4–2.—A summary of the serologic picture of *Coccidioides immitis.*

if the titer levels off and then begins to fall, the prognosis is considered to be good. For this disease and, in fact, for all other fungus diseases, the serologic titers may appear to be extremely low when compared with those usually seen with bacterial and viral diseases. This is typical for fungus diseases; in fact, titers as low as 1:4 or 1:8 are never considered too low to be significant when one is dealing with a mycosis. Undoubtedly, what is more important than the actual titer is whether, from repeated tests, the titer remains unchanged, increases or decreases; i.e., the direction that titers take is more important in fungus diseases than the actual number recorded from a given dilution.

If one is uncertain that a given culture is *Coccidioides immitis* or if one has a suspected culture but cannot find arthrospores, a mycelial suspension of the fungus may be inoculated into the peritoneal cavity of mice. Warning: This is a dangerous procedure and should be done only by experienced personnel working under a hood. In 1–2 weeks, mice develop coccidioidomycosis. Upon autopsy, one observes numerous, hard white lesions lining the peritoneal cavity and/or infecting almost any organ. One- to two-millimeter pieces from these infected areas are cut out, placed on a microscope slide with 1–2 drops of 10–20% KOH and heated gently; a coverslip is added. In many instances, this procedure may be difficult because the nodules may be very hard. It may be necessary to cut or tease apart the nodules and let the material set in the KOH for half an hour or so before observing it microscopically. Using the high-power lens, one observes numerous spherules containing endospores. Again, the endospores are 5 microns in diameter, but as they mature up to the spherule size of 80 microns (even up to 200 microns in mice), one sees the various intermediate stages and sizes.

Therapy

In the disseminated form, coccidioidomycosis is a difficult disease to manage. In many instances, the prognosis is grave. Amphotericin B is considered by many to be the drug of choice, but there is really not much choice. It is about the only antibiotic currently available with which there has been success; however, amphotericin B is a rather toxic drug and must be administered slowly and carefully.

Slides

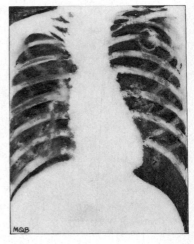

Slide 4–1.—This is a chest film showing an excavated thin-walled nodule of coccidioidomycosis in the left apex. Occasionally, tumors mimic this appearance.

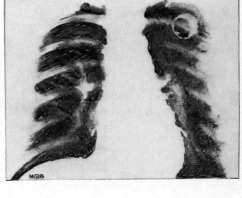

Slide 4–2.—This is a tomogram of the same patient to better demonstrate the thin-wall excavated nodule of coccidioidomycosis. Often these nodules appear as "ring" shadows that are perfectly round and not irregular as shown here.

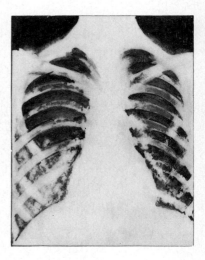

Slide 4–3.—In this film multiple nodular changes are seen in the lung fields with a predominance in the right lower lung field. These nodules may excavate and form thin-walled cysts. This nodulation is characteristic of fungal granulomatous disease which, in this case, is coccidioidomycosis.

The first three slides show radiographs of patients with coccidioidomycosis. This disease usually presents with systemic involvement; however, in some instances dermal manifestation may be evident. Such lesions take on various forms so that there is no *typical* dermal lesion for this disease. The following are examples of dermal lesions from patients with coccidioidomycosis; observe the great variety in the appearance and location.

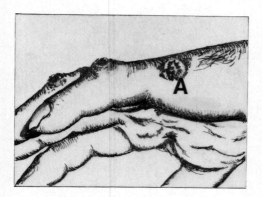

Slide 4–4. — Note the small lesion on the left hand (A). Nothing about the appearance of this lesion leads one to suspect that it is caused by a fungus. If such a lesion is to be examined for the possibility of a pathogenic fungus, first surface decontaminate the area with 70% alcohol. Then remove some material from the edge of the lesion; divide this material into halves, part of it to be used to culture for fungi and the remainder to be used in direct microscopic examination. Place one portion of this material on a microscope slide with 1–2 drops of 10–20% KOH, heat gently, add a coverslip, press down gently on the coverslip and then examine, using the high dry magnification lens of the microscope. If such preparations are positive for *Coccidioides immitis,* spherules or sporangia containing endospores or sporangiospores are observed.

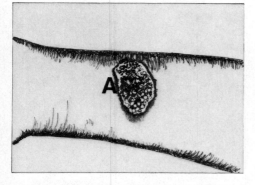

Slide 4–5. — This is another lesion (A) seen on the patient whose hand was shown in Slide 4–4. Again, there is nothing particularly characteristic about this lesion that would lead one to believe that the patient has any fungus disease. Follow the same procedures recommended in the description for Slide 4–4.

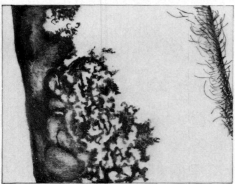

Slide 4–6. — Grossly, this appears to be quite a different lesion than those shown in Slides 4–4 and 4–5; however, this is another example of a patient with coccidioidomycosis.

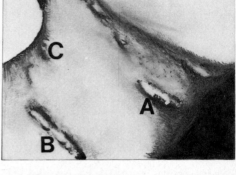

Slide 4–7.—This is another patient with coccidioidomycosis; note the multiple lesions on the neck (A,B,C).

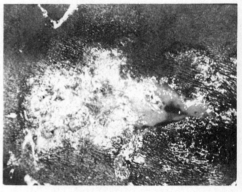

Slide 4–8.—Still another type of dermal manifestation seen in a patient with coccidioidomycosis. This type of lesion may drain; if so, one should be able to see spherules and endospores in direct examination preparations of this material.

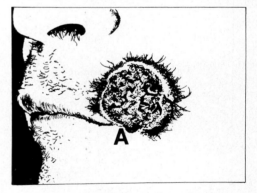

Slide 4–9.—Another example of a cutaneous lesion in a patient with coccidioidomycosis (A).

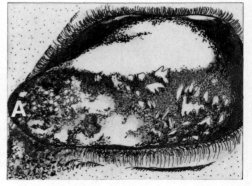

Slide 4–10.—This unusual lesion (A) at the end of the tongue yielded the organism *Coccidioides immitis.*

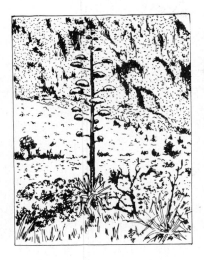

Slide 4–11.—This is not the type of picture of California that the Chamber of Commerce would like to have released. However, despite all the beautiful publicity pictures of that wonderful state, there is a rather large area that is desert. This picture vividly shows the desert country in the southwestern United States and is a good example of a so-called Lower Sonoran Life Zone: very little rainfall, extremely high temperatures in the summer and very little vegetation. This is where the pathogenic fungus *Coccidioides immitis* resides. From certain soils of this type, one is able to isolate thousands of viable particles per gram. Other areas in the world which have similar appearances and conditions should be examined for the presence of this dangerous pathogen.

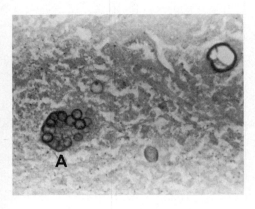

Slide 4–12.—This is how *Coccidioides immitis* appears in human tissue. In the center of the slide is a rather spherical structure (A) which is referred to as the sporangium or spherule. Note that inside the spherule one can see about 15 to 20 well-differentiated endospores. Aside from the disease rhinosporidiosis (in which sporangia may be 300 microns in diameter), no other fungus appears in human tissue in this manner. The hollow spherical structure, off to the side, is a sporangium, but all the internal contents dropped out during staining. This is not unusual.

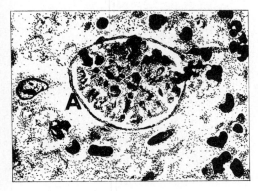

Slide 4–13.—This is another example of *Coccidioides immitis* as it appears in human tissue. The large structure in the middle of this slide is a spherule (A) which contains numerous endospores.

Slide 4–14.—This is a photomicrograph of a PAS stain of human tissue infected with *Coccidioides immitis*. In this slide are at least 3 mature spherules (A, B,C), which stain a pink color with the PAS stain. Inside these structures, one can begin to see the development of the endospores. Throughout this tissue, one can also see several other PAS-positive structures representing endospores in various stages of development, leading up to mature spherules. This slide is very characteristic for coccidioidomycosis.

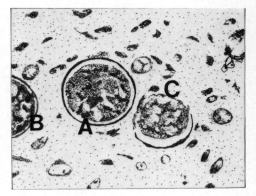

Slide 4–15.—There are at least 8 mature spherules (reddish-purple circular structures) in this slide from a human case of coccidioidomycosis. These spherules are mature, so they are filled with endospores.

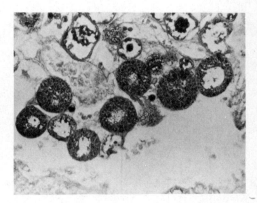

Slide 4–16.—Animals can be infected with *Coccidioides immitis*. Experimentally, we most frequently use the mouse. However, the guinea pig is also a suitable animal. Note the large masses of firm, rough, lobulated nodules being held between the forceps (A). All of this tissue is packed solid with the spherules of *Coccidioides immitis*. To examine this material, cut out very small pieces (1–2 millimeters in diameter) and place them on a microscope slide. Tease this tissue apart, or even mascerate it, add 1–2 drops of 10–20% KOH, heat gently, add a coverslip, press down on it firmly and examine microscopically for the fungus.

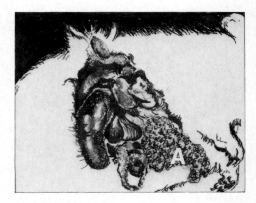

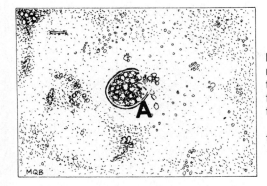

Slide 4–17.—This is an example of how *Coccidioides immitis* appears in direct examination preparations. This particular examination was done on sputum from an infected patient. In the middle of this slide one can discern a spherule (20–30 microns in diameter) which contains numerous endospores.

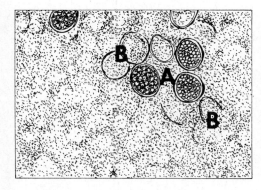

Slide 4–18.—This is a direct examination preparation of material from an animal infected with *Coccidioides immitis.* For this preparation we used tissue from an infected mouse; however, the organism appears in an identical fashion in human tissue. In the center of this slide (A) are 5 or 6 spherules. At least 2 of them are very mature because they are filled with endospores. Also one can see 3 or 4 spherules (B) which developed to maturity and then broke open, releasing endospores into the surrounding tissue.

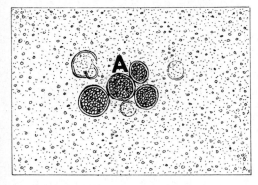

Slide 4–19.—This is a direct examination preparation of human tissue. In the center of this slide are 6 or 7 sporangia showing various stages of development (A).

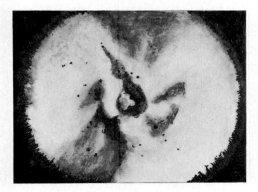

Slide 4–20.—This is the fungus *Coccidioides immitis* as it appears on Sabouraud's agar after 3–4 weeks' incubation at room temperature. It is a very innocent-looking white culture; however, this is the highly infectious state of this fungus. Most isolates of *C. immitis* look like this. The underside of the colony is slightly tan to a darker color.

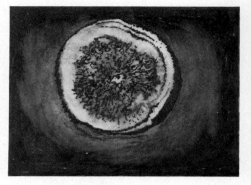

Slide 4–21.—This is a more unusual isolate of *Coccidioides immitis* grown on Sabouraud's agar at room temperature for 2–4 weeks. The culture has some gray color; cultures of this fungus are not *always* a pure white color.

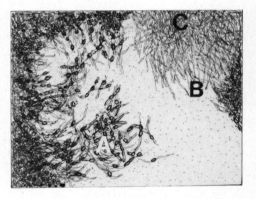

Slide 4–22.—If one takes small portions from the room temperature (or 35–37 C) cultures of *Coccidioides immitis* shown in Slide 4–21, and examines them microscopically in lactophenol cotton blue preparations, one sees what is shown in this slide, namely, large masses of hyphae of which some seem to be a little coarser and have taken up more of the cotton blue dye (A). These areas contain numerous infectious arthrospores. Most people have the impression that the entire culture of *Coccidioides immitis* converts into arthrospores. This is not true. In this slide are many hyphae that have not produced arthrospores (B,C). In fact, in many cultures it is not unusual to have to search a microscope slide for a considerable period of time before one sees the characteristic arthrospores.

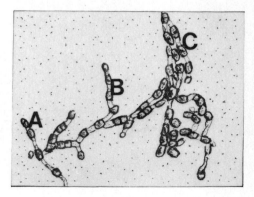

Slide 4–23.—This is a higher magnification of the central field seen in Slide 4–22. Several pieces of hyphae have converted into the characteristic arthrospores. Note the barrel-shaped appearance of alternate cells; these are the arthrospores (A,B,C).

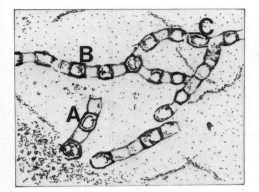

Slide 4–24. — This is a high-magnification photomicrograph of the arthrospores of *Coccidioides immitis* as they grow in either soil or laboratory cultures. Note that it appears that every other cell in the hyphae has converted to arthrospores (A,B,C). These individual cells are highly infectious. This is the outstanding microscopic feature of *Coccidioides immitis* when it is grown on Sabouraud's agar and incubated for 1–4 weeks. No other pathogenic fungi form structures that can be confused with these.

HISTOPLASMOSIS

Synonym

Darling's disease.

Definition and Clinical Forms

As with coccidioidomycosis, there may be numerous clinical forms of histoplasmosis. I have elected to describe this disease in three clinical forms.

PRIMARY ACUTE. — After inhalation of infectious particles, individuals may be asymptomatic or may develop flu-like symptoms and experience chest pain, shortness of breath and hoarseness. After a week or two the symptoms disappear. Radiologically, diffuse or discrete lung lesions may or may not develop. When such lesions are present, they always calcify eventually.

The outstanding feature of the primary acute form of histoplasmosis is the fact that all such individuals become skin test positive. In major endemic areas between 70% and 95% of all residents are skin test positive. Thus, in some areas in the world this is a very common disease. In North America it is *the* most common cause of lung calcification.

CHRONIC CAVITARY. — In this form of the disease relatively large pulmonary lesions develop. For unknown reasons the body is able usually to contain such lesions. These lesions may exist in a relatively quiescent state, causing the patient little problem or discomfort, or they may progress to disseminated histoplasmosis. This clinical form is often mistaken for tuberculosis.

SEVERE DISSEMINATED. — Fortunately, only a small percentage of persons infected with this fungus progress into this clinical form. In this state, histoplasmosis is a disease of the reticuloendothelial system, and, as such, any organ may be involved. When massive dissemination occurs, histoplasmosis is often fatal.

Etiology

Only one fungus causes the disease histoplasmosis, namely, *Histoplasma capsulatum*. This name was derived from several sources: the "histo" refers to the fact that the fungus is frequently found in histiocytes; "plasma" refers to the early, erroneous concept that the etiologic agent was a protozoan; "capsulatum" refers to the erroneous conclusion that the organism has a capsule in vivo.

The perfect (i.e., sexual) stage is called *Emmonsiella capsulata*.

Epidemiology

Until the 1960s it was believed that there was only one endemic area in the world for histoplasmosis. This region included a rather large area in the eastern United States, sometimes referred to as the Mississippi River Valley Basin (Fig 4–3). Today we still recognize that this is the major endemic area; however, we also know that histoplasmosis is found in virtually every part of the world.

The fungus *Histoplasma capsulatum* resides exclusively in soil and especially in soil containing the feces of certain birds. In the United States, the feces of starlings, chickens and bats are most frequently implicated. It is relatively easy to isolate this organism from old chicken houses or from city parks where large numbers of birds have resided for several years.

This organism lives in soil in the mycelial form and produces microaleuriospores, which are the infectious particles. These spores are small and light enough to be carried by wind currents and enter the lung milieu.

Predilections

As with most other fungus diseases, little is known about predisposing factors for histoplasmosis. It appears that almost any individual converts to skin test positive after being exposed to the infectious particles. However, the real question is, why do only certain individuals progress into the disseminated form of histoplasmosis? In a few instances, exposure to massive numbers of infectious particles may overwhelm the body's defense mechanisms, resulting in a more severe form of histoplasmosis; however, such exposures have not been recorded in all individuals with the disseminated state, which leaves many questions as yet unanswered.

Tissue Form and Histopathology

Although this fungus produces septate hyphae and spores while growing in soil, it grows in a completely different state inside the human body. In vivo, it grows as relatively small (3–5 microns in diameter), nonencapsulated, intra-

Fig 4–3. — Major endemic area for histoplasmosis in the United States (> 60% population are skin test positive).

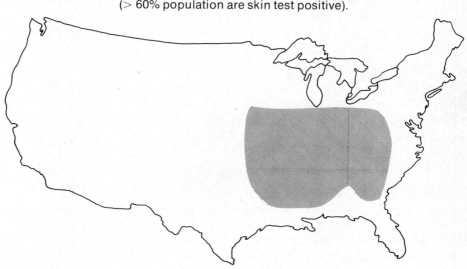

cellular yeast cells. They are the smallest yeast cells and of the major fungus diseases they are the only ones that grow intracellularly.

Suspected tissue may be stained with H&E; however, the PAS stain is more specific for all fungi. In such preparations, it is not unusual to see 20–40 small yeast cells growing intracellularly. In this regard, the in vivo form of *H. capsulatum* is similar to what one sees with *Leishmania* species. Another stain which is extremely helpful is methenamine silver (GMS).

Very often when the yeast cells of *Histoplasma capsulatum* are fixed, the cytoplasm has a tendency to shrink away from the cell wall. When stained, the cytoplasm takes up more of the dye; thus the area between the cytoplasm and the cell wall gives the impression of being clear. This common observation led earlier investigators to believe, erroneously, that this yeast cell had a thin capsule surrounding it.

Direct Microscopic Examination

With most of the other fungus diseases I have recommended the use of KOH preparations to observe the organism. In histoplasmosis, however, it is extremely difficult to be certain if one is observing this fungus because the yeast cells are so small, lack characteristic features, usually are intracellular and often are mistaken for air bubbles or fat droplets. For this reason, I recommend that suspected tissue or sputum be streaked onto a microscope slide, allowed to air dry and stained with either Wright or Giemsa stains. In such preparations one observes relatively small yeast cells (3–5 microns in diameter) either intra- or extracellularly. Regarding this point, there are two important features.

1. Although histoplasmosis is an intracellular disease, it is *not* uncommon, especially in smeared preparations, to observe this organism extracellularly.
2. This yeast cell, like all other fungi, is somewhat reluctant to retain as much of gram stain as do bacteria. Thus, gram-positive fungi (and all fungi are gram-positive, although a better term might be gram-dubious) tend to exhibit a speckled effect as opposed to being uniformly gram-positive. This "gram-reluctance" makes it a little more difficult to observe gram-stained fungi in tissue until one has had some experience. This is why I recommend the Wright or Giemsa stains.

Culture

Histoplasma capsulatum is a true dimorphic fungus; it can be grown in the mycelial form at room temperature and as a true yeast at 35–37 C.

Materials for culturing may be sputum, biopsy material, or blood; if available, bone marrow and adrenals are the best. Such materials should be cultured on Sabouraud's agar (or Mycosel or Mycobiotic media) at room temperature and brain-heart infusion agar at 35–37 C. Although this sounds quite simple, in many instances it is difficult to culture this organism, even from widely disseminated cases. The reason for this problem is unknown. However, sometimes it is possible to overcome the problem by inoculating 5–10 milliliters of blood into 100–200 milliliters of brain-heart infusion broth and incubating it at 35–37 C.

Grown on Sabouraud's medium at room temperature, *H. capsulatum* develops in 1–4 weeks as a white or tan, very fluffy fungus. The underside of the colony may be brown. Microscopically, one observes masses of clear, septate, small hyphae, microaleuriospores (so called because they are relatively small, 3–5 microns) and the larger, diagnostically important, tuberculated macro-aleuriospores. The latter structures are 10–20 microns in diameter and have a very thick wall which may be smooth; however, most often they are covered with numerous bumps or spines (tubercles) which are 2–3 microns in diameter. The relatively large, tuberculated macroaleuriospore is the outstanding diagnostic feature of this organism when it is grown at room temperature.

When *H. capsulatum* is cultured at 35–37 C, it does not produce hyphae or spores; one cultures yeast only. The colony usually develops in 1–3 weeks as a white to slightly tan, smooth, typical appearing yeast colony. Microscopically, one observes numerous yeast cells, 3–5 microns in diameter. It is not uncommon to observe some hyphae in colonies which have been grown as yeast for the first time. These are remnants from the room temperature form and disappear upon repeated subculturing of the yeast at 35–37 C. There is nothing particularly characteristic about the yeast cells except their relatively small size and the fact that, when they are subcultured onto Sabouraud's agar and incubated at room temperature, the mycelial fungus grows out once again.

Occasionally, one encounters strains of *H. capsulatum* that do not produce macroaleuriospores—or any that are produced lack the characteristic tubercles or have an unusual morphology. In such instances, conversion to the yeast form normally is considered sufficient to establish identification. However, some workers like to inoculate a heavy mycelial suspension (0.5 milliliters) into the peritoneal cavity of mice. One to 3 weeks later they sacrifice these animals and examine and culture the organs.

The filamentous form of this fungus is dangerous to work with in the laboratory. In this state, the highly infectious microaleuriospores are produced. Physicians should inform laboratory personnel that they may be culturing *H. capsulatum,* and laboratory workers should culture potentially infected material in slants instead of Petri dishes. Microscopic preparations of the filamentous form of this fungus should be made only by experienced personnel working under a hood. The yeast form of this fungus is *not* a laboratory hazard.

Other Laboratory Tests

In histoplasmosis, serologic information is of great value diagnostically, prognostically and therapeutically. Man is so exquisitely sensitive to the skin test material histoplasmin that in some instances it is even necessary to dilute it. This material reacts very well in individuals exposed to the organism, and cross-reactivity is not a great problem. Unfortunately it may interfere with other serologic tests and therefore is not recommended in suspected cases. As with coccidioidomycosis, the precipitin titer begins to rise shortly after exposure to the organism; however, this test is not nearly so reliable or consistent as it is in patients with coccidioidomycosis. As a precipitin titer disappears, complement-fixing (CF) antibodies begin to appear. CF titers may exist for several years even after a clinical cure. Once again it should be emphasized that antibody titers for mycoses are extremely low when compared to the titers seen in bacterial or viral diseases. More important than the dilution titer is whether one observes a rise or a fall in a given titer. A continuously rising titer indicates increased dissemination and a bad prognosis, and may indicate to the physician that the particular therapy he is using has not taken effect; stable or decreasing titers are a good sign.

There is considerable current research in the area of serologic methods for histoplasmosis, e.g., a double diffusion test using histoplasmin. It is hoped that some of these new, more reliable, and more informative tests will become commercially available in the near future.

Therapy

In disseminated histoplasmosis, amphotericin B is the drug of choice. The cure rate is not very high; however, for the present, this rather toxic antibiotic is about the only available treatment.

African Histoplasmosis

In recent years a disease known as African histoplasmosis has been reported from Africa. Most commonly this disease localizes in skin, lymph nodes and bone. Subcutaneous abscesses and skin lesions may be oberved. As yet, we know very little about this disease. Medical personnel in tropical and subtropical areas should be alerted that it may exist in their area of the world.

In vivo, the fungus produces relatively large yeast cells (7–15 microns in diameter) which are found inside giant cells.

The etiologic agent of this disease is *Histoplasma capsulatum* var. *duboisii*. It can be grown in a filamentous state on Sabouraud's agar (with or without antibiotics) at room temperature. Grossly and microscopically the culture resembles *H. capsulatum,* i.e., it develops tuberculate macroaleuriospores and microaleuriospores; however, these may take several weeks to develop. On brain-heart infusion agar (35–37 C) a yeast colony is formed. Initially, the yeast cells may be small, but eventually they become 7–15 microns in diameter.

Slides

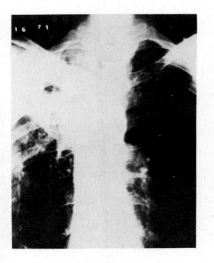

Slide 4–25. — This radiograph shows retraction of the superior mediastinum toward the right apex and an elevation of the right hilus. This indicates fibrosis and scarring in a chronic disease. Multiple cavitary lesions are seen in the right apex indicating active granulomatous disease, which in this case is histoplasmosis.

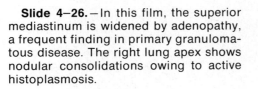

Slide 4–26.—In this film, the superior mediastinum is widened by adenopathy, a frequent finding in primary granulomatous disease. The right lung apex shows nodular consolidations owing to active histoplasmosis.

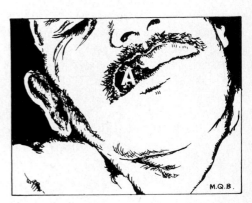

Slide 4–27.—This is a patient with histoplasmosis. Note the lesion on the right side of his upper lip (A). Dermal lesions are rarely seen in patients with this fungus disease; when they are seen, they are not particularly characteristic.

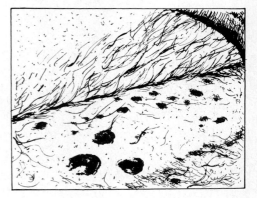

Slide 4–28.—This is a patient with disseminated histoplasmosis. Note the rash-like lesions. Again, dermal lesions are rarely seen in this mycosis.

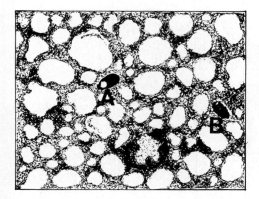

Slide 4–29.—This is a gram stain of tissue infected with *Histoplasma capsulatum.* In this slide are 2 prominently stained yeast cells (A,B). These are gram-positive yeast cells of *H. capsulatum;* note the usual manner in which these yeast cells have retained gram stain. In particular, 1 cell, near the edge of the picture, has the "blotchy" effect previously mentioned.

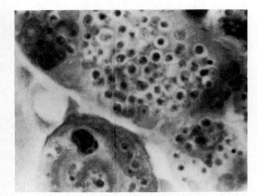

Slide 4–30.—This photomicrograph clearly demonstrates the intracellular nature of *H. capsulatum.* The larger of the infected cells probably contains in excess of 40–50 yeast cells.

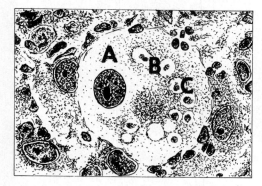

Slide 4–31.—This is another picture of how *Histoplasma capsulatum* appears in a stained section of tissue. Note that the giant cell (A) in the middle of the slide contains at least 8 yeast cells (B,C) in focus. Also, note that these yeast cells appear to be surrounded by clear capsules; this is a fixation artifact.

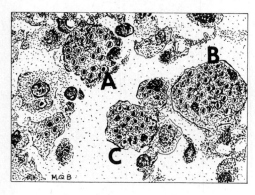

Slide 4–32.—Note how the macrophages (A,B,C) in this tissue section have engorged themselves with yeast cells of *Histoplasma capsulatum.* These cells contain so many yeast cells that it is impossible to count them. In heavily infected areas, this is a typical picture.

Slide 4–33.—This is a Giemsa-stained smear from a nose ulcer in which the intracellular cells of *Histoplasma capsulatum* (A, B) can be seen readily, especially in the cell near the middle of the field.

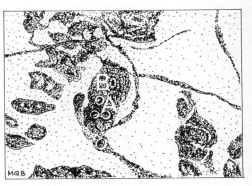

Slide 4–34.—This is a tissue section stained with methenamine silver (GMS) from a patient with histoplasmosis. In such preparations, the yeast cells retain the silver and appear black. Thus all of the spherical black particles throughout the slide are yeast cells of *H. capsulatum*. Although this stain may not be used routinely in many laboratories, if the time and facilities are available, it is an extremely valuable stain for all of the mycoses.

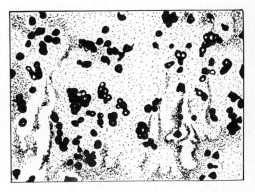

Slide 4–35.—This is a typical appearing culture of *Histoplasma capsulatum* grown on Sabouraud's agar at room temperature for 2–4 weeks. The fungus colony is white and very fluffy. The underside of this colony is a light tan color. This photograph is a good example of the gross, room temperature, colonial morphology of *Histoplasma capsulatum*. This highly infectious organism should not be grown in large bottles or Petri dishes.

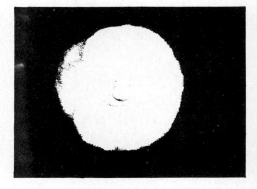

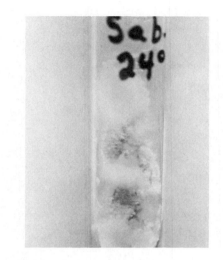

Slide 4–36.—This is the safest way to grow *Histoplasma capsulatum* at room temperature, namely, *in test tubes* containing Sabouraud's agar. The colony is white to buff-brown, and fluffy in appearance.

This organism, *Coccidioides immitis* and *Blastomyces dermatitidis* usually produce white, fluffy colonies when grown on Sabouraud's agar and incubated at room temperature. All 3 fungi are laboratory hazards when cultured at room temperature. All of them (and these are the only 3 to worry about) usually produce nonpigmented colonies. Beware of the white, fluffy colonies.

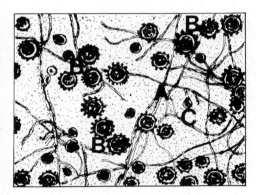

Slide 4–37.—This is a photomicrograph of *Histoplasma capsulatum* grown on Sabouraud's agar and incubated at room temperature. In the background are the septate hyphae (A). However, the characteristic structures, with which this fungus are identified, are the tuberculated macroaleuriospores (B). This slide is filled with these characteristic spores. In some places on this slide a few of the infectious microaleuriospores (C) are visible.

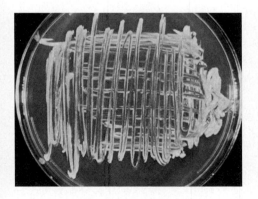

Slide 4–38.—This shows the colonies that *Histoplasma capsulatum* forms when cultured on brain-heart infusion agar and incubated for 1–2 weeks at 35–37 C. Notice how remarkably different this form is from the room temperature colony. These colonies look like the colonies of many other yeast cells; in fact, they could readily be mistaken for many bacterial colonies. Grossly, these colonies differ from bacterial colonies only in that yeast colonies grow much more slowly. Usually the yeast form colonies of *H. capsulatum* are off-white to a light tan color. Other than these features, such colonies are not particularly helpful in identifying this fungus, except by proving that the organism is a dimorphic fungus.

Slide 4–39.—This is a gram stain of *Histoplasma capsulatum* cultured on brain-heart infusion agar, incubated at 35–37 C. These yeast cells (A,B,C) are relatively small, 3–5 microns in diameter, and have few characteristic features. It is not unusual to see a few hyphal elements in such preparations, especially when this is the first time that the hyphal form has been converted to the yeast form. This yeast does not reproduce with a broad-based bud and lacks a capsule.

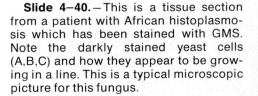

Slide 4–40.—This is a tissue section from a patient with African histoplasmosis which has been stained with GMS. Note the darkly stained yeast cells (A,B,C) and how they appear to be growing in a line. This is a typical microscopic picture for this fungus.

Slide 4–41.—This is a higher magnification of the fungus *Histoplasma capsulatum* var. *duboisii*. This is a smear from an infected mouse spleen, and the typical appearing yeast cell is the relatively clear structure in the middle of the field (A). Note that this yeast cell looks very similar to the yeast cells of *Blastomyces dermatitidis*.

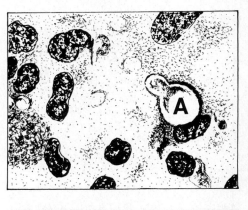

Slide 4–42.—This is another tissue section from a patient with African histoplasmosis. In the center of this slide are approximately half a dozen yeast cells of *H. capsulatum* var. *duboisii* (A,B,C).

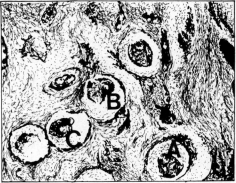

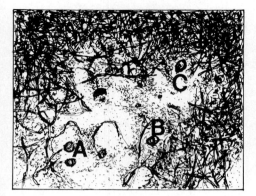

Slide 4–43. — This is a photomicrograph of *H. capsulatum* var. *duboisii* cultured on Sabouraud's agar and incubated at room temperature. Note the abundance of hyphae; however, macroaleuriospores are beginning to develop (A,B,C). It is not unusual for 2 months to elapse before the macroaleuriospores begin to appear.

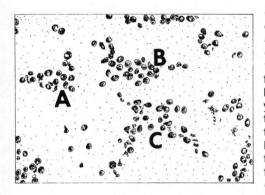

Slide 4–44. — This is a photomicrograph of *Histoplasma capsulatum* var. *duboisii* cultured on brain-heart infusion agar at 35–37 C. This organism is a true dimorphic fungus, having converted from the room temperature filamentous form into a yeast form when cultured on brain-heart infusion at 35–37 C. These yeast cells (A,B,C) are a great deal larger than those of *H. capsulatum.* Other than that, they have no characteristic features. If some of these yeast cells are subcultured on Sabouraud's agar and incubated for 1–2 weeks at room temperature, the growth of the filamentous form of this fungus will be observed.

SELF-EVALUATION QUESTIONS
(Answers at end of questions)

Check the ONE best answer for each question:
1. Coccidioidomycosis and histoplasmosis are contracted from infected
   a. _____ pigeons
   b. _____ soil
   c. _____ humans
   d. _____ bats
2. After exposure to *Coccidioides immitis* an individual becomes skin test positive in
   a. _____ 1–6 days
   b. _____ 7–28 days
   c. _____ 30–60 days
   d. _____ 60–100 days
3. In coccidioidomycosis, which of the following is a poor prognostic sign?
   a. _____ conversion to skin test positive
   b. _____ positive precipitin titer
   c. _____ decreased precipitin titer
   d. _____ increasing complement fixation titers

4. The major endemic area in the world for coccidioidomycosis is
   a. _____ southwestern United States
   b. _____ the Sahara Desert
   c. _____ the Mississippi River Valley Basin
   d. _____ Argentina
5. In tissue, *Coccidioides immitis* is seen most often as
   a. _____ septate hyphae
   b. _____ coenocytic hyphae
   c. _____ spherules and endospores
   d. _____ intracellular yeast
6. Arthrospores are the infectious particles of
   a. _____ *Histoplasma capsulatum*
   b. _____ *Coccidioides immitis*
   c. _____ both of the above
   d. _____ *Blastomyces dermatitidis*
7. Which of the following diseases is the major cause of lung calcification in the U.S. today?
   a. _____ sporotrichosis
   b. _____ coccidioidomycoses
   c. _____ nocardiosis
   d. _____ histoplasmosis
8. The infectious particle of *Histoplasma capsulatum* is the
   a. _____ microaleuriospores
   b. _____ macroaleuriospores
   c. _____ yeast
   d. _____ septate hyphae
9. A unique feature of histoplasmosis is
   a. _____ encapsulated yeast
   b. _____ coenocytic hyphae
   c. _____ granules containing yeast cells
   d. _____ intracellular yeast
10. Grown on brain-heart infusion agar at 35 C, *Histoplasma capsulatum* produces
   a. _____ yeast cells
   b. _____ tuberculate macroaleuriospores
   c. _____ the infectious microaleuriospores
   d. _____ encapsulated yeast cells

For the following questions, fill in the blanks:

11. Approximately _____ million people in the U.S. have, or have had, histoplasmosis or coccidioidomycosis.
12. When a patient with coccidioidomycosis converts from skin test positive to negative, the prognosis is usually _____.
13. The infectious particles of *Coccidioides immitis* are the _____.
14. The drug of choice for patients with coccidioidomycosis is _____.
15. The chronic cavitary form of histoplasmosis is often mistaken for _____.
16. The name of the species of the fungus causing histoplasmosis was given because early investigators erroneously believed that, in vivo, the fungus had a _____.

17. Some of the best tissues to examine for *Histoplasma capsulatum* are

    _____ .

18. The outstanding microscopic feature of *Histoplasma capsulatum* cultured at room temperature is the _____ .

19. The etiologic agent of African histoplasmosis is _____ .

20. African histoplasmosis appears to be a disease of _____ areas of the world.

Answers to questions 1–20.

1. b	11. 50 to 60
2. b	12. bad (grave)
3. d	13. arthrospores
4. a	14. amphotericin B
5. c	15. tuberculosis
6. b	16. capsule
7. d	17. bone marrow and adrenals
8. a	18. tuberculated macroaleuriospores
9. d	19. *Histoplasma capsulatum* var. *duboisii*
10. a	20. tropical

5 / Dermatophytoses

Synonyms

Ringworm, athlete's foot, jock itch, dermatomycoses.

Background

Historically, a dermatophyte was the first microorganism that was proved to cause a disease of humans (1839). At that time, and during the ensuing 50 to 75 years, little attention was paid to such diseases and their etiologic agents. After all, why should a physician get excited about a case of athlete's foot when an epidemic of plague was raging in the nearby village?

Eventually, two groups of scientists began working independently on the dermatophytoses. Unfortunately, these two groups developed their own systems of terminology for these diseases. To this day, these different terminology systems are used; however, during the past decade the two groups have begun to cooperate.

Initially, the dermatologists described these diseases by the body area; e.g., tinea capitis meant a ringworm infection of the scalp, tinea barbae referred to the beard, tinea corporis referred to the body, tinea pedis referred to the foot. On the other hand, the mycologists felt more comfortable referring to the scientific name of the etiologic agent, paying little attention to the clinical picture and site of infection. The compromise over these different forms of terminology is to name the disease by the body area and to designate the specific etiologic agent, e.g., tinea barbae owing to *Microsporum gypseum*.

Definition

The term dermatophytoses refers to infections of the skin, nails or hair that are caused by fungi classified as dermatophytes. Normally, it is not considered that dermatophytic fungi can cause systemic disease; in fact, with only one minor exception, none of these fungi can grow at 37 C.

Epidemiology

The dermatophytic fungi include numerous species of fungi which are contained in three major genera. These organisms occur worldwide, mainly in soil and on certain animals. Within a given locale one never sees all of these organisms causing disease; the most one usually sees in a given area is six to eight species.

The dermatophytoses are some of the most common diseases of man. Although incidences of infection vary greatly, at least 10–20% of the world's population may be infected with these organisms. Most investigators believe that these diseases are acquired exogenously; however, because they can be isolated from such a high percentage of the world's population and in many instances individuals show no clinical evidence of disease, many of these fungi might some day be considered part of man's flora.

An outstanding feature of these organisms is that they are all keratinophilic, which means that they love keratin. This knowledge has resulted in a rather interesting method for isolating dermatophytic fungi from soil. This procedure is known as "hair baiting." Place some soil in a sterile Petri dish. Add enough sterile water to dampen the soil. Obtain some human hair (clippings from the local barber will suffice), wash the clippings with acetone or ether to remove the fat and oils, let dry and cut into 1-centimeter pieces. Sterilize (e.g., autoclave) this hair and sprinkle it onto the moistened soil in the Petri dish. Place the cover back on the Petri dish and incubate for 2–3 weeks. During this period it may be necessary to add a little more water to keep the soil moist. Because dermatophytic fungi are keratinophilic, they grow on hair. Thus, if keratinophilic fungi are present in the soil sample, they will grow onto the shafts of the hair. (Grossly, one observes numerous white tufts of hyphae growing on the hair shafts.) Infected pieces of hair may then be removed and cultured for identification of the specific fungus. This isolation method has helped elucidate the epidemiology of many of these fungi.

Clinical Forms

Before discussing the specific etiologic agents, general clinical features of these diseases and ways to identify some of the more important etiologic agents will be pointed out.

First of all, let us look at the tissues they invade:

HAIR. — Infected hair often appears dry and lacking in luster. If it breaks off, it may leave bald areas. Often, the scalp is dry and scaly; in some instances, elevated lesions may form. Of all the etiologic agents, only two are considered to be infectious, namely, *Microsporum audouinii,* a common cause of "epidemic" ringworm of the scalp in children, and *Trichophyton tonsurans,* which causes tinea capitis in adults.

Hair infections are classified according to the manner in which the fungus invades the hair. Some species of dermatophytes grow only on the *outside* of the hair shaft; this type of infection is called "ectothrix." On the other hand, certain other species of dermatophytes invade only the *inside* of the hair; this type of hair infection is called "endothrix." By determining if a given infection is either endothrix or ectothrix, one can begin to get an indication of a possible etiologic agent.

Another phenomenon associated with hair infections that tends to give a preliminary clue regarding the specific etiologic agent is the fact that several of the infecting fungi fluoresce when the hair is examined with a Wood's or black light (an ultraviolet light with maximum emission at 3,660 angstroms). This type of examination should be done routinely in suspected cases of tinea capitis. If fluorescing hairs are observed, they should be removed for direct examination preparations and culturing.

NAILS. — Although several nails on either the hands or the feet may be infected, it is unusual for all of them to appear infected. In many instances, the infected nails look chalky and dull. Frequently, the nail is raised, with debris and keratinized cells underneath it. Nail infections are most often caused by organisms that belong to the genus *Trichophyton;* however, some investigators believe that *Candida albicans,* a yeast and not a dermatophyte, causes a relatively high percentage of the nail infections that are thought to be caused by dermatophytes.

The important point about nail infections is that, *regardless* of the etiologic agent, one only observes hyaline, septate hyphae in nail tissue. It is impossible to know the specific etiologic agent without first obtaining a pure culture.

Nail infections caused by dermatophytes evolve very slowly; i.e., several weeks to months to years may pass as the disease develops.

SKIN. — Initially, small isolated lesions may appear on any part of the body. These lesions evolve very slowly but may eventually cover large areas of the body. Some of the etiologic agents (especially those contracted from another human) induce little inflammation. On the other hand, dermatophytes that spread from animal to man may cause considerable inflammation. Regardless of the etiologic agent, one observes hyaline, septate hyphae only in skin.

Identification

On the subject of identification, there are two schools of thought:

1. Before therapy is initiated, one need only be certain that a fungus is the source of a given patient's problem. Confirmation of this suspicion is usually made with a direct microscopic examination of potentially infected tissue.
2. It is important to identify a specific etiologic agent because in some instances the therapeutic regimen is affected and information of this type is of value epidemiologically. (Being a mycologist, I tend to favor the latter point of view.)

Identification of dermatophytes is done with the following parameters:

1. *Clinical picture.* This has already been covered and will be gone into again in greater detail when specific etiologic agents are discussed. However, I cannot overemphasize the slowly evolving nature of ringworm infections.
2. *Wood's light.* Hair infections should be examined with this procedure. If positive results are obtained, this may be the first evidence that a fungus is involved; however, if no fluorescence is observed, this does not rule out the possibility of a fungus infection as many do not fluoresce.
3. *Direct examination.* Remove skin, hair or nails from the infected area and place them on a microscope slide to which 1–2 drops of 10–20% of KOH are added. Place a coverslip on this preparation, heat gently and then press down on the coverslip. Examine, using the high dry lens of the microscope. With potentially infected hair, try to determine if the fungus is growing endothrix or ectothrix. In examining skin or nail material, look for hyaline, septate hyphae. Because nail tissue is very hard, to obtain a good direct microscopic examination preparation it may be necessary to let the pieces of nail incubate for half an hour to an hour in KOH.
4. *Culture.* For hair, skin and nail cultures use Mycosel or Mycobiotic medium and incubate at room temperature. If the patient has a skin infection, remove flakes of skin from the edge of the lesion. If contamination might be a problem, surface decontaminate *briefly* with 70% alcohol. In dealing with infected nails, clip small portions from the infected area and force the nail clippings down into the medium.

Regardless of the etiologic agent involved, most dermatophytic fungi grow very slowly. A 1- to 3-week incubation period may be required before the first growth of the colony is observed.

In the study of dermatophytoses it is not unusual to encounter a very strange phenomenon known as the "Id" reaction. One may observe skin lesions on a patient, but all attempts to culture dermatophytic fungi from these lesions are negative; however, one still may believe that a dermatophyte is involved. If this is true, the reaction is called an "Id" or dermatophytid. Supposedly, these are sterile lesions which have been induced by an active lesion, dermatophytic in origin, on another area or part of the body quite distant from the "Id" reaction. Thus, in such instances, one should investigate other areas of the body to see if dermatophytes are present. To date, this phenomenon is a mystery, but mycologists believe it exists.

Therapy

The greatest breakthrough in this field came a few years ago with the development of the antibiotic griseofulvin. This is truly a wonder drug and undoubtedly has resulted in the successful cure of millions of patients with dermatophytoses. However, this drug does present some problems:

1. It is fungistatic, not fungicidal; this means that it must be given until the infected tissue sloughs off the still viable etiologic agent.
2. It must be taken orally on a regular basis and usually for extended periods of time.
3. This antibiotic can be expensive if taken, as indicated in most cases, for the prescribed 2–3 months.
4. The percentage of cures for long-standing ringworm infections of the nails, and especially of toenails, is extremely low.

Usually griseofulvin is recommended when the patient has large areas of involvement or when other therapeutic agents have failed.

For the treatment of smaller, localized lesions we now fortunately have clotrimazole and miconazole at our disposal. These recently developed drugs are becoming available in most areas of the world. They are sold under various trade names as creams or ointments. Both of these agents are very effective in the treatment of dermatophytoses and are of such a broad spectrum that they are also very effective against most of the so-called superficial mycoses. These agents are gaining rapid acceptance for the treatment of localized lesions.

In many parts of the world, Castellani's paint is still held in high regard, especially since it is relatively inexpensive and quite effective for cases of tinea corporis. For tinea cruris and tinea interdigitales, Whitfield's ointment, an old standby, is still recommended by many physicians. It must be remembered that in many areas in which dermatophytoses are more common and severe than in the United States, drugs such as griseofulvin, clotrimazole and miconazole are out of the financial reach of the majority of the population. This is why the older treatments are still being used.

I would like to make a special comment about cases of ringworm of the foot. True, many of the above-mentioned drugs are effective, but one should also try to eliminate some of the conditions which enhance the growth of the dermatophytic fungi on the feet and toenails. The patient should do everything possible to keep his feet dry by frequently changing socks and applying powders. The feet should be scrubbed thoroughly daily and dried with a coarse towel. The latter treatment aids in the sloughing of infected tissue. One may be able to eradicate a fungus from infected feet temporarily; however, if the patient persists in maintaining his feet in a greenhouse atmosphere, the disease soon reappears.

Mycology

All of the agents of dermatophytoses are listed in three genera: *Microsporum, Epidermophyton* and *Trichophyton.* All of these organisms should be cultured on Sabouraud's agar with antibiotics (Mycosel or Mycobiotic) and cultured for several weeks at room temperature. None of these organisms is dimorphic. Very few biochemical identification procedures are available for the dermatophytes; thus, identification is based on the gross and microscopic morphology of the colony. Depending upon the author, spores on dermatophytic fungi are called either conidia or aleuriospores.*

MICROSPORUM. — Species of the genus *Microsporum* infect hair and skin only. In hair, usually an ectothrix infection results.

M. audouinii. — Before the advent of griseofulvin, this organism was a common cause of epidemic ringworm of the scalp in school-age children. This is one of the few fungi that can be readily transmitted from one person to another. This organism is anthropophilic, which means that it always resides on man.

It is rarely found in soil or on animals other than man. Infected hair fluoresces with Wood's light.

M. audouinii forms a white, fluffy colony after 1–2 weeks' incubation at room temperature. The underside of the colony is a pale yellow to light orange color.

Microscopically, the organism rarely produces spores although terminal chlamydospores may be observed.

Some persons confirm suspicions of *M. audouinii* by inoculating it into test tubes containing a few grains of moistened, sterilized rice. This is one of the few dermatophytes that will not grow on this substrate. The organism occurs worldwide.

M. canis. — This organism causes sporadic outbreaks of hair and skin infections worldwide. The organism is mainly zoophilic, which means that it is usually found on animals other than man; however, it occasionally spreads from these animals to cause infections in man. Erythema is common in the lesions caused by *M. canis.*

The colony of *M. canis* is white and fluffy. Sometimes the rich canary yellow color on the bottom of the colony shows through the white, fluffy mycelium on the top.

Microscopically, *M. canis* is characterized by the formation of large, thick-walled, warty, spindle-shaped macroaleuriospores, which contain 8–12 septa. Such structures are characteristic and are the major way to identify this organism.

M. ferrugineum. — In many ways, this organism is similar to *M. audouinii.* In certain areas of the world this is a common cause of tinea capitis. It is anthro-

---

*Many authors call the spores "conidia." If an organism produces both large and small spores, they are called macroconidia and microconidia, respectively. Technically speaking, spores of dermatophytes should be called aleuriospores. If an organism produces both large and small aleuriospores, they are called macroaleuriospores and microaleuriospores, respectively.

philic and causes infected hairs to fluoresce. This organism is relatively un-common in the Americas but is seen quite often in Asia, Africa and Europe. This fungus causes an ectothrix infection in hair.

Most authorities believe that *M. ferrugineum* occurs in two colonial forms: (1) a very slow-growing, wrinkled, suede-like, yellow- to rust-colored colony or (2) a more rapid-growing colony which is usually flat, leathery and white. However, in some strains different colors develop in various sectors of the colony, especially upon original isolation.

Microscopically, there are few structures of any diagnostic value. Occasion-ally the septate hyphae appear to have exceptionally thick septa, giving the impression of "bamboo" hyphae.

M. gypseum. — This organism is considered to be geophilic (which means that it resides in soil). With the hair baiting method, this organism has been isolated from almost every soil in the world. Fortunately, this organism is not a common cause of ringworm infections in man. Sporadically it has been re-ported to cause hair and skin infections, especially tinea barbae. This organ-ism causes ectothrix infections. Infected hairs do not fluoresce.

The colony of *M. gypseum* is flat, light brown (cinnamon color) and very powdery in appearance. Occasionally, throughout the colony, numerous small white tufts of hyphae appear; these are so-called pleomorphic areas, which in mycology means that no spores are being formed on the hyphae, i.e., they are devoid of reproductive structures.

Microscopically, *M. gypseum* forms thin-walled, spindle-shaped aleurio-spores which contain 4–6 septa. These aleuriospores are extremely charac-teristic of *M. gypseum* and are one of the main diagnostic features.

EPIDERMOPHYTON. — Strangely, this genus contains only a single species. This fungus attacks skin and nails only.

E. floccosum. — As far as is known today, this fungus infects only man and thus is anthropophilic. *E. floccosum* is worldwide in distribution and in some areas is a common cause of infections of the groin, body, feet and nails.

The colony of *E. floccosum* is usually a yellow to greenish (olive drab) color and is quite wrinkled or folded. The colony has a very fine, fuzzy texture, almost like suede leather. As with *Microsporum gypseum*, this organism commonly has areas of pleomorphism.

Microscopically, the colony forms characteristic club-shaped aleuriospores. These spores are usually formed singly or in clumps of 2 or 3. The cell wall of the aleuriospore is smooth. The spore contains 2–3 septa, and the end of it is quite blunt or rounded. This organism forms no microaleuriospores.

TRICHOPHYTON. — Species belonging to the genus *Trichophyton* may attack skin, hair or nails. Hair infected with these organisms does not fluoresce. *Trichophyton* species infect man and other animals. In many areas of the world they are a major concern because feet and nail infections caused by some of the species of *Trichophyton* are extremely difficult, if not impossible, to cure.

These organisms rarely form macroaleuriospores, thus making identifica-tion more difficult. Microscopically, many of them form microaleuriospores and produce hyphae in spiral forms and other strange structures, which to some authorities are taxonomically important.

T. tonsurans. — This organism is anthropophilic and is worldwide, although major endemic areas are North and Central America, northern Europe, Southeast Asia and many of the South Pacific Islands. The organism causes endothrix hair infections in which the inside of the entire hair shaft seems to be filled with spores. This type of hair infection causes the hair either to burst open or to grow in a coil in the stratum corneum. These coils of hair are grossly visible and are referred to as "black dot" tinea capitis. *T. tonsurans* may cause tinea corporis, tinea pedis and occasionally onychomycosis. Some people refer to this organism as the etiologic agent of "adult ringworm of the scalp"; this disease form is considered to be quite contagious. Infected hairs do not fluoresce.

Colonies of *T. tonsurans* look powdery and are a yellow to reddish brown color. The underside of the colonies is a rich red to brown color. Colonies often have a suede appearance, i.e., short, aerial hyphae with many wrinkles and folds.

Microscopically, *T. tonsurans* forms an abundance of microaleuriospores which are usually club-shaped and borne directly on the hyphae. As some of the microaleuriospores mature, they enlarge further and look like miniature balloons. Many forms of *T. tonsurans* grow better with thiamine added into the medium, thus helping to separate them from *T. mentagrophytes* and *T. rubrum.*

T. violaceum. — The disease that this organism induces is very similar to that seen with *T. tonsurans.* Most often, *T. violaceum* causes scalp infections (e.g., "black dot" ringworm), although tinea corporis and nail infections are not uncommon. Endothrix hair infections are formed, and, as with *T. tonsurans,* the entire hair shaft becomes filled with spores. The major difference between *T. tonsurans* and *T. violaceum* is the geographic distribution pattern. *T. violaceum* is rarely seen in the Americas; however, it is quite common throughout North Africa, the Mediterranean area, Russia, China, India and Southeast Asia.

T. violaceum is anthropophilic. When hair is infected, it does not fluoresce.

In culture, *T. violaceum* is quite distinctive because it forms a very wrinkled, heaped up, waxy colony which is a purple-red color. As the colony gets older, or when it is subcultured, it begins to produce white, aerial hyphae.

Neither microaleuriospores nor macroaleuriospores are produced by this fungus. The hyphae are a mass of tubes that grow in all directions and look rather mixed up and distorted.

In this chapter it has been possible to cover only a few of the etiologic agents of the dermatophytoses. A textbook on this subject is available.*

---

*Rebell, G., and Taplin, D.: *Dermatophytes, Their Recognition and Identification* (Coral Gables, Fla.: University of Miami Press, 1974).

Slides

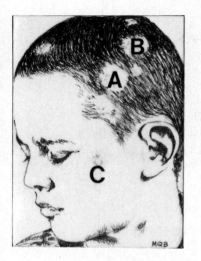

Slide 5–1. — This is an example of a child with tinea capitis. Note the bald areas on the head (A,B) and the lesions spreading down to his cheek (C). This infection developed over a period of several weeks and responded very well to griseofulvin.

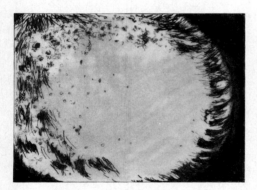

Slide 5–2. — This is another case of tinea capitis. Note how different it is from that shown in Slide 5–1. A large area of the scalp has been involved, a considerable amount of hair has been lost, and the tissue is responding in a rather violent fashion to this particular etiologic agent.

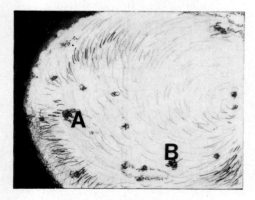

Slide 5–3. — This is a case of tinea capitis characterized by the formation of scutula, (saucer-shaped crusty lesions) (A,B) on the scalp.

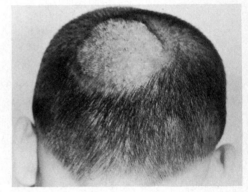

Slide 5–4.—This shaved head shows vividly the extent of this particular scalp infection. Note the considerable amount of erythema in the lesions.

Slide 5–5.—In this case of tinea capitis only a solitary, well-defined, nonerythematous lesion is seen.

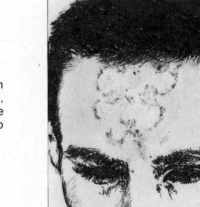

Slide 5–6.—This is a case of ringworm on the forehead. In this particular case, there was no involvement of the hair. The lesions took several weeks to develop to this state.

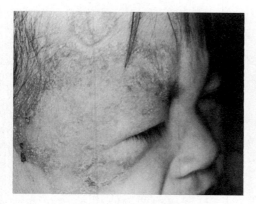

Slide 5–7.—In KOH preparations from the edge of the large lesion we saw numerous, septate, hyaline hyphae. Skin scrapings were planted into Mycosel agar. Two weeks later we identified the etiologic agent as *T. tonsurans.* Similar clinical pictures caused by this organism are frequently seen in the Orient and Pacific islands.

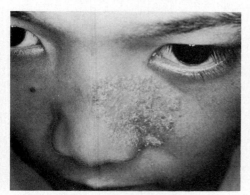

Slide 5–8.—This patient (and the one in Slide 5–7) is from the Philippines. Upon culture we identified the etiologic agent as *M. gypseum.* In the Republic of the Philippines this organism is not an uncommon cause of tinea corporis.

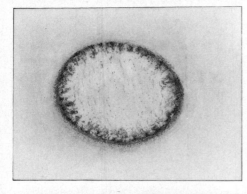

Slide 5–9.—This is a single, isolated lesion in a case of tinea corporis. This lesion took 2–3 weeks to develop to this size. In this case, as well as all other cases involving nails or skin, material can be scraped from the lesion and examined for hyaline, septate hyphae in direct examination preparations with KOH.

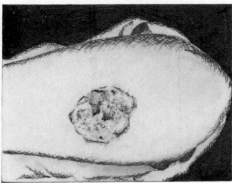

Slide 5–10.—This is a case of tinea corporis of the arm. No other lesions were observed. This lesion took 4–5 weeks to develop to this size.

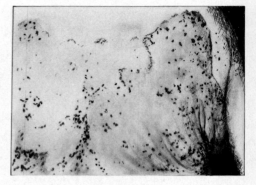

Slide 5–11.—This is a generalized case of tinea corporis caused by *Trichophyton rubrum*. Perhaps this case became so extensive because the patient had an underlying immunologic deficiency.

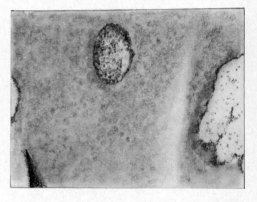

Slide 5–12.—This is another example of a case of tinea corporis.

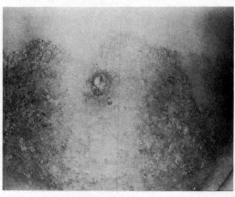

Slide 5–13.—This long-standing, slowly evolving infection of the stomach area was caused by *T. rubrum*.

Slide 5–14.—This is a rather typical case of tinea cruris caused by *Trichophyton rubrum*.

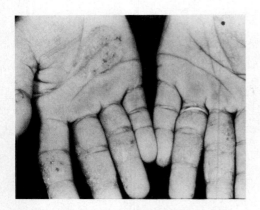

Slide 5–15.—The palms of the hands and the fingers are infected with a dermatophyte.

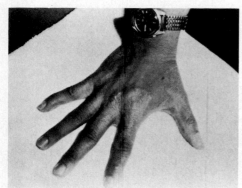

Slide 5–16.—This is another case of a dermatophytic infection of the hand.

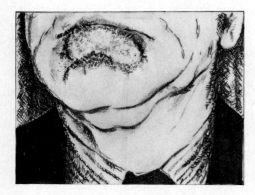

Slide 5–17.—This is a case of tinea barbae caused by *Trichophyton mentagrophytes.* Initially, very small lesions developed on the chin in the area where a beard would grow. These lesions developed slowly, eventually coalesced and, after 2–3 months, resulted in what is seen here.

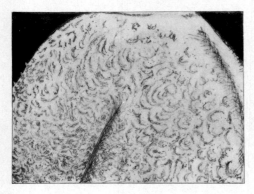

Slide 5–18.—This unusual clinical manifestation of tinea corporis is called tinea imbricata. Note the circular, almost snake-like appearance of these lesions over the entire body. Tinea imbricata is a special form of tinea corporis caused by the dermatophyte *Trichophyton concentricum.*

Slide 5–19. — This is the arm of the patient who was shown in Slide 5–18. This strange disease affects thousands of native peoples throughout Southeast Asia and the Pacific islands.

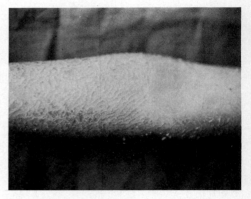

Slide 5–20. — This is an example of a case of tinea pedis. The lesion took several months to develop to this size. Without appropriate therapy, it would continue to develop in this patient over a period of several months or years.

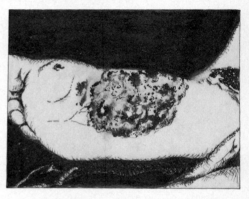

Slide 5–21. — This is a case of tinea unguium or onychomycosis, probably caused by *Trichophyton rubrum.* Note how all the nails are involved except one (A). This patient has had this infection for several years. The chances of curing it, even with griseofulvin, are poor.

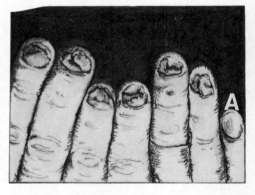

Slide 5–22. — This picture of a mouse infected experimentally with *Trichophyton mentagrophytes* shows how an animal, other than man, appears when infected with a dermatophyte.

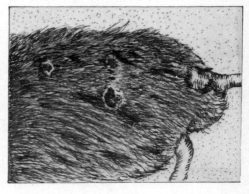

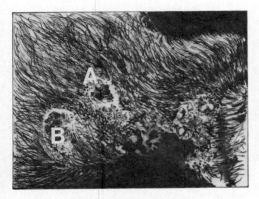

Slide 5–23.—This is a higher magnification of the lesions (A,B) seen in the animal in Slide 5–22. Occasionally, dermatophytic infections can be a severe problem in a research animal colony.

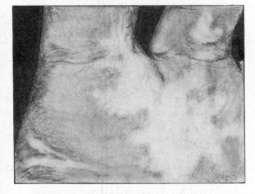

Slide 5–24.—This rather unusual picture shows skin eruptions caused by griseofulvin. They occurred shortly after this individual began taking griseofulvin and developed to such an extent that he was forced to discontinue the medication. Fortunately, cases of this type are extremely rare.

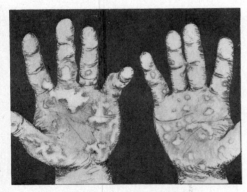

Slide 5–25.—This is a lower magnification of the individual seen in Slide 5–24. This shows the extent of the griseofulvin allergy manifested by the patient. Several days after he stopped taking griseofulvin, his hands returned to normal.

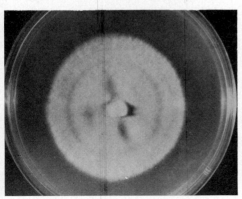

Slide 5–26.—This is a picture of the top of a culture of *Microsporum audouinii*. A white, fluffy colony is typical for this organism. As with all dermatophytic fungi, growth is slow. This colony took 3–4 weeks to attain this size. The underside of this culture is a yellow to orange color.

Slide 5–27.—This is very typical of a young culture (1–2 weeks old) of *Microsporum canis*. The canary yellow color on the underside of the colony is so intense that it can often be seen through the white, fluffy, aerial hyphae on the surface.

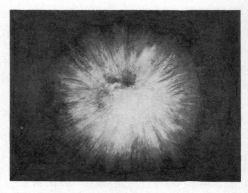

Slide 5–28.—This is a typical culture of *Microsporum ferrugineum*. In some of the older textbooks, this organism was classified in the genus *Trichophyton*. This colony's intense orange color suggested the species name *ferrugineum*. This organism rarely forms aerial hyphae on primary isolation; it is usually flat and very wrinkled.

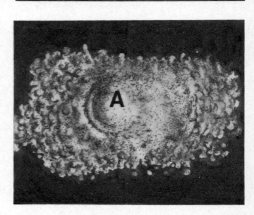

Slide 5–29.—This is a culture of *Microsporum gypseum*. The colony is a light brown color and powdery in appearance. In the center of the colony, one can begin to see the development of white tufts of hyphae; this is a pleomorphic area (A), and no spores will be formed here.

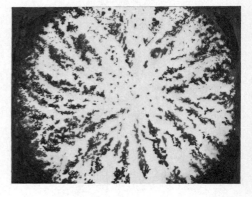

Slide 5–30.—This is a slightly different type of isolate of *Microsporum gypseum;* however, it still is light brown, flat and powdery.

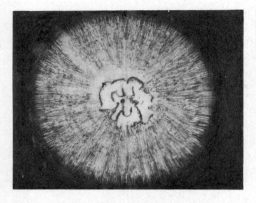

Slide 5–31. — This is the organism *Epidermophyton floccosum.* This particular colony is several weeks old. In culture, *E. floccosum* is usually a yellow to green to brown color, forms a rather flat colony and may rapidly develop areas of pleomorphism.

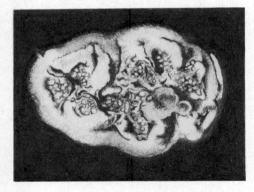

Slide 5–32. — This is another isolate of *E. floccosum.* Although this organism produces an abundance of hyphae, it rarely becomes fluffy unless areas of pleomorphism develop.

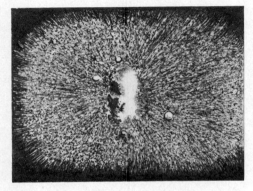

Slide 5–33. — This is the organism *Trichophyton concentricum.* This colony took 3–5 weeks to develop to this size; it is white, lacks an abundance of aerial hyphae and is very wrinkled and heaped up.

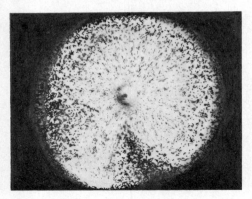

Slide 5–34. — This is the granular form of *Trichophyton mentagrophytes.* This organism also takes a downy cultural form in which an abundance of white, fluffy mycelium predominates in the culture.

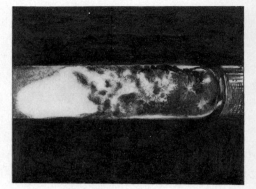

Slide 5–35. — This is the underside of a culture of *T. mentagrophytes;* it is an intense yellow to orange color. On occasions this color becomes brown to reddish, making it difficult to distinguish the organism from *T. rubrum.*

The next 4 slides are examples of different cultural forms of the dermatophyte *Trichophyton rubrum.* This is a very important fungus throughout the world, and it is worthwhile to be able to recognize the various types of colonies it forms.

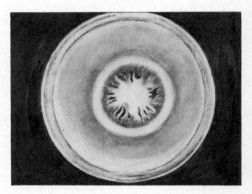

Slide 5–36. — This is a colony of *T. rubrum* after 2–4 weeks' incubation on Mycosel agar at room temperature. The colony is not particularly fluffy, it is very wrinkled and slow-growing, and the red pigment on the underside can be seen through the top of the colony.

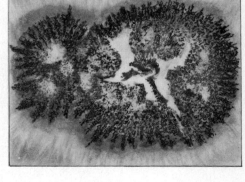

Slide 5–37. — This is an excellent example of the granular form of *T. rubrum.* Note the lack of white aerial hyphae. This colony develops very slowly, is quite compact and wrinkled and grows close to the medium.

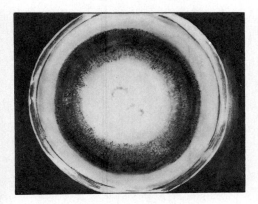

Slide 5–38.—This is a "downy" isolate of *T. rubrum.* The top side of the colony is white and fluffy, while the underside has an intense red pigment.

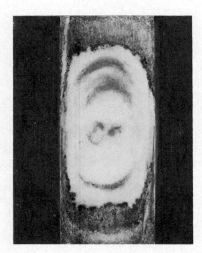

Slide 5–39.—This is another example of the "downy" form of *T. rubrum.* This culture contains an abundance of white, fluffy mycelium on the top of the colony. The underside of the colony is a dark red color.

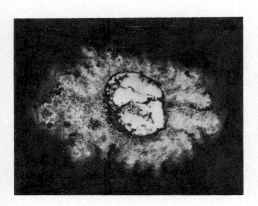

Slide 5–40.—This is a culture of *Trichophyton schoenleinii* grown for 4–6 weeks at room temperature on Mycosel agar. This particular isolate has formed few aerial hyphae; in fact, most of the hyphae are growing under the surface of the medium.

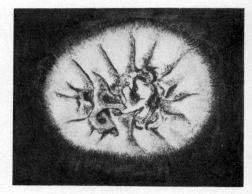

Slide 5–41.—This is another isolate of *T. schoenleinii*. This culture is composed of white aerial hyphae and has many wrinkles. Note that the center is heaped up.

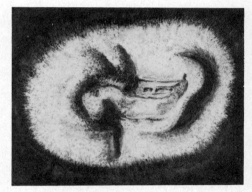

Slide 5–42.—This is a colony of *T. tonsurans*. This colony usually is a tan color and is quite wrinkled.

Slide 5–43.—This is a culture of *T. violaceum*. The species name was derived from the violet color of the colony.

The following are some photomicrographs showing the distinguishing microscopic features of some of the dermatophytes.

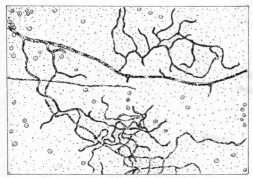

Slide 5-44.—This is a typical picture showing the mycelium of *Microsporum audouinii*. Spores are rarely seen; only hyphae are visible in this slide.

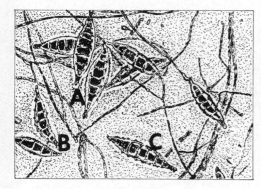

Slide 5-45.—This is a typical photomicrograph showing the characteristic macroaleuriospores (A,B,C) of *Microsporum canis.* Surrounding these spores is what appears to be a halo of light because this photograph was taken with a phase microscope. These macroaleuriospores are relatively large, have thick, rough walls and tapered ends and usually contain 8-12 septa at maturity.

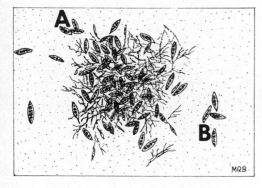

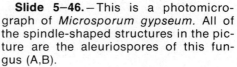

Slide 5-46.—This is a photomicrograph of *Microsporum gypseum.* All of the spindle-shaped structures in the picture are the aleuriospores of this fungus (A,B).

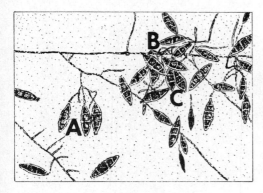

Slide 5-47.—This is a higher magnification of the characteristic spores of *M. gypseum.* These aleuriospores (A,B,C) are spindle-shaped and have thin walls and 2-5 septa.

Slide 5–48.—This is a photomicrograph of the aleuriospores of *Epidermophyton floccosum.* Usually these aleuriospores (A,B) are borne in pairs, contain 2–5 septa and have blunt ends.

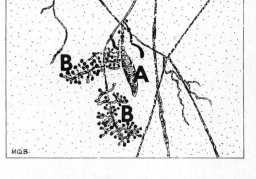

Slide 5–49.—This is a characteristic photomicrograph of the fungus *Trichophyton mentagrophytes.* The large, dark structure in the middle of this picture (A) is a macroaleuriospore; such spores are rarely seen in cultures of *T. mentagrophytes.* The bunches of smaller particles in this picture, next to the macroaleuriospore, are the microaleuriospores (B), which are borne "en grappe." These spores are spherical to elongated, and the "en grappe" arrangement is characteristic of this organism.

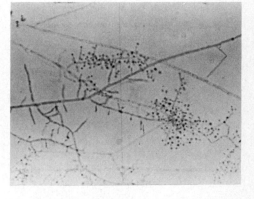

Slide 5–50.—This is another photomicrograph of *T. mentagrophytes.* Again, note the grape-like clusters of small, spherical spores (microaleuriospores).

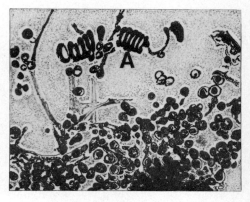

Slide 5–51.—This is another photomicrograph of *T. mentagrophytes* in which we see coiled-up hyphae; these are frequently referred to as spiral hyphae (A). This type of formation is seen in several of the *Trichophyton* species; therefore, it is not diagnostic for a given organism.

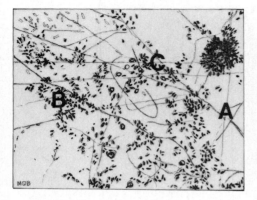

Slide 5–52.—This is a photomicrograph of the dermatophyte *T. rubrum*. In the background are hyphae (A). All of the small masses (B,C) throughout this entire picture are the microaleuriospores. Usually the spores are spherical to elongated and are borne directly on the hyphae; however, occasionally they occur in rather large clumps, giving the erroneous impression that they are borne "en grappe" (i.e., as seen in *T. mentagrophytes*).

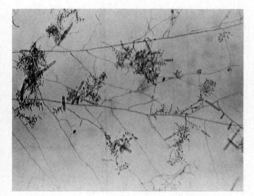

Slide 5–53.—This is a photomicrograph of *T. tonsurans*. Numerous clusters of microaleuriospores can be seen. Occasional macroaleuriospores can also be seen.

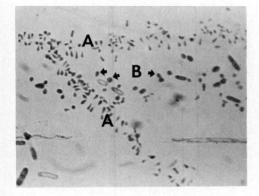

Slide 5–54.—This is a higher magnification of a culture of *T. tonsurans*. A few macroaleuriospores are evident, as are numerous typical microaleuriospores (A). Some of the microaleuriospores appear to have swollen up into balloon-like spores (B), which are characteristic of this organism.

Slides 5–55 to 5–59 illustrate the difference between endothrix and ectothrix infections of hair.

Slide 5–55.—This is an excellent example of an ectothrix infection. The dark mass (A) consists of spores growing on the outside of the hair shaft. Note that these spores seem to form a mosaic pattern.

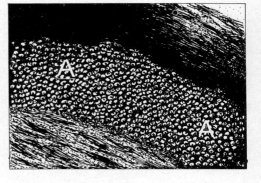

Slide 5–56.—This also is an ectothrix infection, but the photograph was taken from the top, looking down on the hair, to show the mosaic pattern of the spores (A) growing on the outside of the hair shaft. The hair shaft is the lighter area in the central portion of the picture (B).

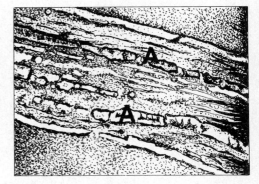

Slide 5–57.—This is an excellent example of an endothrix infection. The hair shaft takes up the majority of the picture, going from left to right across the slide. Inside the hair shaft septate hyphae (A) are growing. This is one form of an endothrix hair infection.

Slide 5–58.—This also is an endothrix infection; however, this particular fungus produces spores (A) instead of hyphae inside the hair shaft.

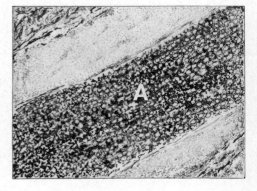

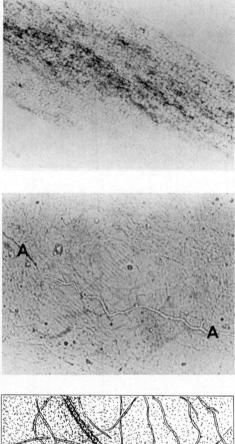

Slide 5–59.—This is another example of an endothrix infection in which the entire hair shaft has become filled with spores. This is typical of the type of invasion seen in the so-called black dot infections. *T. tonsurans* was cultured from this case.

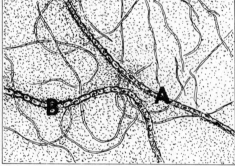

Slide 5–60.—This is a KOH-positive preparation of skin (or nails). (This means that dermatophytic organisms have been seen in the tissue.) Observe the slender hypha which goes from one side of the field to the other (A). In this slide a micrometer has been superimposed. This is a very simple device which can be inserted into the eyepiece of any microscope. When calibrated (with each of the lenses) it is a simple matter to measure cells and hyphae. The micrometer is a valuable tool in medical mycology because size is such an important factor.

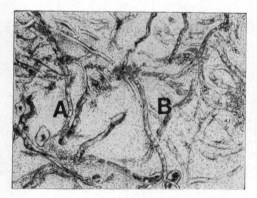

Slide 5–61.—This is a higher magnification of a dermatophyte growing in skin or nail tissue. It is a little easier to see the long, slender strands of hyphae (A,B) in this photomicrograph.

Slide 5–62.—This is a photomicrograph of a PAS preparation of skin containing a dermatophyte. This type of preparation is rarely made but readily demonstrates the presence of the hyphae (A,B).

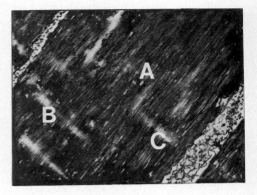

Slide 5–63.—This is a positive hair penetration test, which means that the organism can be identified as *Trichophyton mentagrophytes*. The dark areas in this slide are the hair (A). Note the burrowing effect of this fungus, i.e., the V-shaped wedges (B,C) in the hair shaft. Remember that this is an in vitro test and has no relationship to the way this organism grows in vivo.

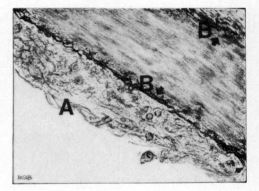

Slide 5–64.—In contrast to Slide 5–63, this is how *T. rubrum* appears when growing in the hair penetration test. Note that no burrowing or V-shaped wedges can be seen; the fungus simply grows as septate hyphae (A) on the outside of the hair shaft (B). This is an excellent test to distinguish between *T. mentagrophytes* and *T. rubrum*. The only drawback is that it takes 2–3 weeks to complete. For this reason some workers culture these organisms on urea agar; in 2 days most strains of *T. mentagrophytes* are positive (i.e., turn the medium red) and most strains of *T. rubrum* are negative.

SELF-EVALUATION QUESTIONS
(Answers at end of questions)

Check the ONE best answer for each question:

1. Ringworm infections of the scalp are called
   a. _____ onychomycosis
   b. _____ tinea capitis
   c. _____ tinea pedis
   d. _____ tinea barbae
2. Dermatophytic infections may be acquired from
   a. _____ soil
   b. _____ fellow man
   c. _____ other animals
   d. _____ all of the above
3. The hair baiting procedure depends on the fact that all dermatophytes
   a. _____ grow on hair
   b. _____ are keratinophilic
   c. _____ reside in soil
   d. _____ grow at 25 C.

4. Which of the following may cause epidemic ringworm of the scalp?
   a. _____ *Microsporum audouinii*
   b. _____ *M. canis*
   c. _____ *M. gypseum*
   d. _____ *Trichophyton rubrum*
5. In nails infected with a *Trichophyton* species, one would expect to see
   a. _____ septate hyphae and macroaleuriospores
   b. _____ coenocytic hyphae and microaleuriospores
   c. _____ septate hyphae and microaleuriospores
   d. _____ hyaline, septate hyphae
6. The antibiotic griseofulvin
   a. _____ may be given intravenously
   b. _____ must be taken orally
   c. _____ is fungicidal
   d. _____ is relatively inexpensive
7. The most important parameter used to identify cultures of *Microsporum* species is
   a. _____ gross and microscopic morphology of the colony
   b. _____ arrangement of microaleuriospores
   c. _____ color of colony
   d. _____ biochemical tests
8. Aleuriospores of *Epidermophyton floccosum* are usually produced
   a. _____ in pleomorphic areas
   b. _____ singly on hyphae
   c. _____ in pairs
   d. _____ in sporangia
9. The most reliable method for distinguishing between *Trichophyton rubrum* and *T. mentagrophytes* is
   a. _____ the morphology of microaleuriospores
   b. _____ the morphology of macroaleuriospores
   c. _____ the pigment produced in the mycelia
   d. _____ the hair penetration test
10. A dermatophyte which is anthropophilic grows mainly on (in)
    a. _____ man
    b. _____ other animals
    c. _____ soil
    d. _____ hair

For the following questions, fill in the blanks:

11. In the hair penetration test, _____ _____ grows or burrows into hair, creating V-shaped wedges.
12. When a dermatophyte grows inside the hair shaft, the infection is said to be _____.
13. An "en grappe" arrangement of microaleuriospores is characteristic of

_____ _____.

14. Which one of the *Microsporum* species produces large, thick-walled macroaleuriospores with 8 to 12 septa? _____ _____.
15. When a portion of a fungus colony produces white, sterile (i.e., lacking spores) hyphae, this is called an area of _____.

16. Tinea imbricata, a special form of tinea _____, is caused by _____ _____.
17. As the microaleuriospores of _____ _____ enlarge, they look like miniature balloons.
18. "Bamboo" hyphae is a characteristic of *Microsporum* _____.
19. Griseofulvin is least effective in the treatment of ringworm infections of the _____.
20. Many investigators believe that a relatively high number of fungal nail infections, thought to be caused by *Trichophyton* species, are actually caused by the yeast _____ _____.

Answers to questions 1–20.

1. b
2. d
3. b
4. a
5. d
6. b
7. a
8. c
9. d
10. a

11. *Trichophyton mentagrophytes*
12. endothrix
13. *Trichophyton mentagrophytes*
14. *Microsporum canis*
15. pleomorphism
16. corporis, *Trichophyton concentri-cum*
17. *Trichophyton tonsurans*
18. *ferrugineum*
19. nails (especially toenails)
20. *Candida albicans*

6 / Opportunistic Fungi

ONLY 10 TO 15 YEARS AGO, it was relatively simple to place the fungi which a medical mycologist encountered into two separate categories: pathogens and laboratory contaminants (i.e., saprophytes). Having two well-defined categories simplified one's work; however, these precise boundaries are fading. In recent years, and with increasing frequency, the so-called laboratory contaminants are being reported as etiologic agents of human mycoses. Probably the main reason for such a change is that modern medicine manipulates the host to a greater extent and, in so doing, lowers normal defense mechanisms. These are the conditions under which many of the so-called saprophytic fungi of the past become opportunistic pathogens of the present. Many of the diseases they cause are fatal. Unfortunately, because of numerous problems, many of these diseases are not being diagnosed until the patient reaches the autopsy table. The opportunistic fungi cause great diagnostic and therapeutic problems.

Opportunistic fungi might be defined as those organisms which under normal conditions do not cause disease. This definition should immediately focus attention onto the role of predisposing factors. Because many of these factors (such as therapeutic regimens and surgery) are in the hands of the physician, it behooves him to realize that some of his recommendations and/or procedures may increase the risk of a patient's contracting an opportunistic fungus infection. Also, when such a disease is diagnosed in time, the physician should consider changing treatment plans to improve a patient's normal responsiveness.

More and more examples of opportunistic fungus infections are appearing in the literature. I have selected three diseases to illustrate some of the principles involved. In trying to identify an opportunistic fungus not discussed in this chapter, refer to the six methods by which fungi grow in vivo presented in Chapter 1. Regardless of the fungus encountered, placement of it in one of these six categories should be possible. Even if the etiologic agent cannot be identified specifically, at least it will be obvious whether a mycosis is present. Such information is particularly valuable in medical mycology because many of the therapeutic regimens, whatever the etiologic agent, are similar.

This chapter discusses candidiasis, aspergillosis and phycomycosis (zygomycosis).

CANDIDIASIS

Synonyms

Moniliasis, mycotic vulvovaginitis, thrush, candidosis, *Candida* endocarditis.

Definition

Candidiasis may be defined as an acute or chronic, superficial or disseminated mycosis caused by species of the genus *Candida*. Clinical forms are so diverse that *Candida* species undoubtedly are some of the most versatile of all fungal pathogens, even though many are part of the normal flora of man. Candidiasis can mimic anything from a dermatophytic infection of the skin to tuberculosis.

Because the clinical forms of candidiasis are so diverse and numerous, only a few will be mentioned here.

THRUSH. — This is a disease of oral mucous membranes and is characterized by the formulation of white, creamy patches seen most often on the tongue. The white areas are pure cultures of the fungus. If some of this material is scraped off, the underlying tissue is a bright, fiery red color. Most commonly, thrush covers the entire tongue. This is not an infrequent disease of children.

NAIL INFECTIONS. — *Candida* nail infections simulate ringworm infections. Some authorities believe that many of the so-called dermatophytic infections of nails are actually caused by *Candida* species. The nails become hardened and thickened (but not brittle); they assume a brownish color; usually there is not as much debris underneath the nail as when a dermatophyte is the etiologic agent. These are infections which often last for years.

MYCOTIC VULVOVAGINITIS. — This may be a rather common disease in diabetics, pregnant women and those on birth control pills. The lesions resemble a simple eczematoid dermatitis or may show vesicular pustules or form a gray-white pseudomembrane.

SYSTEMIC CANDIDIASIS. — Unfortunately, *Candida* species may also cause pulmonary disease or endocarditis or become widely disseminated to almost any other body organ. Even the meninges may become involved. In some rare instances, especially in children, a very severe, generalized cutaneous form develops. This is usually seen in individuals with underlying immunologic deficiencies. These forms of candidiasis are frequently fatal.

Etiology

Most authorities recognize more than a dozen *Candida* species which can cause human disease. In most instances, *Candida albicans* is the prime etiologic agent of candidiasis. Unfortunately, this particular species is such a common cause of human disease that people have tired of reporting it in the literature. On the other hand, it is an interesting novelty when one finds a case of candidiasis caused by one of the other species. Because investigators like to report such novelties, the literature has become engorged with reports of candidiasis caused by species other than *C. albicans*. While we should be aware that many *Candida* species cause candidiasis, *C. albicans* is still the most important etiologic agent.

Epidemiology

The interesting thing about *Candida albicans* and several of the other *Candida* species is that they are part of man's normal flora. *Candida albicans* can be isolated from the gastrointestinal tract, vagina and oral areas in normal, healthy individuals. Except for the disease actinomycosis, candidiasis is the only common fungus disease caused by normal flora. This unique aspect immediately suggests predisposing factors as the key to the disease process.

Only in extremely rare instances has *Candida albicans* been reported to occur outside of the human body. As man is worldwide, it follows that *Candida* species can be found everywhere.

Candida species are yeasts which reproduce by budding. Some of the species form hyphae under certain conditions; however, because the hyphae look a bit different (septa seem to constrict the diameter of the hyphae), they are often called pseudo-hyphae or pseudo-mycelium.

Predisposing Factors

The list of predisposing factors for candidiasis is very long. Some of those described in the literature are tuberculosis; cancer; tooth extractions; surgery of any type; diabetes; drug addiction; pregnancy; indwelling catheters; long-term antibiotic or, especially, steroid therapy; numerous as yet undescribed dietary factors; and depressed immunologic responsiveness, either genetically determined or induced. In my opinion, the last is probably the key to *all* predisposing factors.

Tissue Phase and Histopathology

All *Candida* species appear the same when growing in vivo.

The PAS stain is the best for visualizing *Candida* species in histopathology slides. In such preparations, all *Candida* species appear pink. Depending on the source of the tissue, there are varying mixtures of yeast cells and pseudo-hyphae. In the more superficial forms of candidiasis, one sees a predominance of budding yeast cells and few pseudo-hyphae. On the other hand, when a *Candida* species invades internal organs, it forms very few yeast cells, reproducing mostly with pseudo-hyphae. This distinction is very important.

The methenamine silver stain (GMS) is also very valuable for seeing *Candida* in histopathology slides: all *Candida* species (like all fungi) stain brown to black.

Direct Microscopic Examination

In many instances, direct microscopic examination can be extremely valuable, diagnostically, therapeutically and even prognostically.

Because the material to be examined depends on the suspected location of the disease, it may be sputum, skin scrapings, vaginal swabs, biopsy material from any type of organ or, rarely, blood. Regardless of the material, it should be placed immediately on a microscope slide with 1–2 drops of 10–20% KOH. If the material is solid tissue, it may be necessary to tease it apart. Add a microscope coverslip, heat very gently and then press down on the coverslip. Microscopically, one looks for the presence of yeast cells and pseudo-hyphae. None of the other important fungal pathogens produces a combination of yeast cells and hyphae in vivo.

Often, the value of KOH preparations is overlooked in suspected cases of pulmonary candidiasis. If one examines sputum from almost any individual it is not too difficult to see yeast cells. In suspected cases of pulmonary candidiasis the question is whether one is seeing normal flora (*Candida* from the mouth) or a *Candida* species which has invaded the lung. Fortunately, using direct examination procedures, it is possible to separate these two. If a *Candida* species forms mostly yeast cells, it may be oral flora. On the other hand, when *Candida* species invade lung tissue, they form very few yeast cells; they form almost exclusively pseudo-hyphae. Thus, if one observes in direct examination preparations numerous strands of pseudo-hyphae and few yeast cells, it may well indicate that the lung has been invaded. This may be a particularly valuable clue because such preparations are not done routinely. When the material is only cultured, it is impossible to differentiate between oral flora and those which truly originated in the lung.

Culture

Candida species grow well on Sabouraud's medium at either room temperature or 35–37 C. The colonies usually develop in 2–3 days as white, typical yeast colonies. Regardless of the species, most of the colonies appear the same. In vitro, all *Candida* species are considered to be monomorphic, growing as nonencapsulated yeast cells at any temperature.

In microscopic preparations from cultures, all *Candida* species form nonencapsulated budding yeast cells. Occasionally, if one digs deeply into the colony, a few pseudo-hyphae can be seen. This observation may represent a first clue that a *Candida* species has been cultured.

At this point, a yeast has been cultured which is monomorphic in vitro. To

Fig 6–1.—Microscopic observations of yeast, cultured on chlamydospore or cornmeal agar for 24–72 hours at room temperature incubation. **A,** yeast other than *Candida* species: *a,* budding yeast cells. **B,** all species of *Candida* except *C. albicans: a,* yeast cells and hyphae. **C,** *Candida albicans* only: *a,* yeast cells, hyphae and chlamydospores.

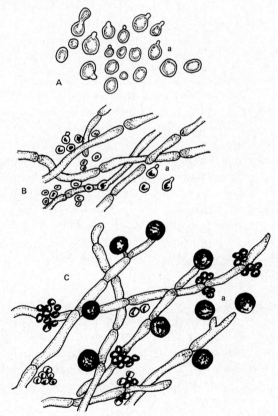

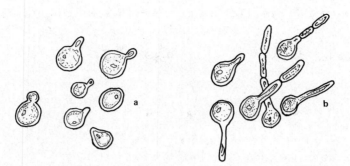

Fig 6–2. — Yeast incubated in serum for 1–2 hours at 35–37 C.
A, most types of yeast. *B, Candida albicans* forming germ tubes.

rule out the possibility of *Cryptococcus neoformans*, do an India ink preparation; *C. neoformans* usually has a capsule, and, in fact, it is the only encapsulated pathogenic yeast. An additional test to separate *Candida* species from
Cryptococcus neoformans is to place the unknown yeast on urea agar. *Candida*
species (except *C. krusei*) do not split urea, but *C. neoformans* does.

There are then several excellent procedures for the identification of *Candida* species. Just recently several commercial laboratories have developed a
battery of assimilation tests which can be done simply and produce results
within 48–72 hours. These tests identify to the species level members of the
following genera: *Candida, Cryptococcus, Geotrichum, Torulopsis, Trichosporon, Rhodotorula* and *Saccharomyces*. Although many of these tests have
become available relatively recently, it appears that they will do much to
revolutionize yeast identification.

An old standby identification method involves the use of chlamydospore or
cornmeal agar. The unknown yeast is either streaked onto or cut into this
medium. If the surface inoculation method is used, place a flamed microscope
coverslip on top of the streaked area. Incubate these plates at either room
temperature or 35–37 C for 24–72 hours, then place the Petri dish directly on
the stage of the microscope and examine the organism. On chlamydospore or
cornmeal agar only members of the genus *Candida* form yeast cells and pseudo-hyphae. In other words, if only yeast cells are seen, then the organism is
not a *Candida* species. If yeast cells and pseudo-hyphae are seen, then the
organism is a *Candida* species. If the organism forms yeast cells, pseudo-hyphae and large chlamydospores, then the organism is *Candida albicans*. This
test has been used for many years to identify *Candida albicans* (Fig. 6-1).

A more rapid presumptive identification method for *C. albicans* is to incubate the unknown yeast in serum at 35–37 C. After 1–2 hours only *C. albicans*
(and many *C. stellatoidea*) forms germ tubes (Fig. 6-2).

Although it is important to proceed as far as possible toward exact identification of an etiologic agent, the really important point is to determine whether
an isolated organism is actually causing a disease process in the patient. I
emphasize this point because in candidiasis we are dealing with organisms
that may be normal flora. Thus it is easy to isolate *Candida* species from an
individual, get carried away with elaborate taxonomic procedures and, in
some instances, become so overly involved that one neglects to prove that the

isolate is the source of the patient's problem. When we are dealing with opportunistic fungi, it is very important that all members of the medical team work together toward a common solution.

Other Laboratory Tests

Currently, considerable research is being done in this area. It is hoped that in the near future some immunologic tests will become available.

Therapy

Because candidiasis represents such a spectrum of clinical entities, it follows that there are several different therapeutic regimens.

For cases of candidiasis without internal organ involvement, the antibiotics nystatin and miconazole are remarkably effective. These drugs usually result in cures for thrush, mycotic vulvovaginitis and many of the superficial skin lesions caused by any of the *Candida* species. The only problem with nystatin is that it cannot be used for systemic infections.

Nail infections caused by *Candida* species are a very difficult problem. The antidermatophytic antibiotic griseofulvin is of no value here. In some instances nystatin helps, especially in cases of paronychia. Over the years, gentian violet has been used with some degree of success. Other older and occasionally effective treatments include sodium caprylate and sodium or calcium propionate. In the Orient many physicians treat *Candida* onychia and paronychia with 1% thymol in chloroform; excellent results are reported. Topical applications of amphotericin B may be of some value, according to certain authors.

In cases of systemic candidiasis, the only drugs which have met with any success are amphotericin B and 5-fluorocytosine.

Again, to emphasize the role of predisposing factors in candidiasis: Removal or correction of such problems may be of as much therapeutic value as some of the aforementioned procedures in achieving a long-lasting cure.

ASPERGILLOSIS

Synonym

None.

Definition

Like candidiasis, aspergillosis may produce numerous clinical pictures. For the present we shall not discuss the allergic forms of this disease but deal only with the frequently fatal disseminated form.

This form of aspergillosis is a granulomatous, necrotizing disease of the lungs which often disseminates hematogenously to various organs. Frequently, this form of the disease is fatal, and, in fact, most diagnoses are presently made at autopsy.

An additional form of aspergillosis is the so-called fungus ball. In this form of the disease, the fungus takes up residence in an old lung cavity. Usually these cavities are the result of old tuberculosis lesions. If the organism remains in these cavities it grows into a huge mass of mycelium, the fungus ball. Radiographically, depending on the position of the patient, these fungus balls may appear to move about.

Etiology

The genus *Aspergillus* is one of the largest of the fungal genera. Hundreds of species have been recorded. To date, 20–30 *Aspergillus* species have been implicated in human disease. The most important are *Aspergillus fumigatus*, *A. flavus* and *A. niger*.

Epidemiology

Aspergillus species are found worldwide. These organisms normally reside as saprophytes in soil. Because they produce trillions of spores which are readily carried into the air, one can isolate various *Aspergillus* species from the air almost any place in the world. This means that man is constantly exposed to spores of *Aspergillus* species.

Predisposing Factors

As we are all constantly exposed to *Aspergillus* species, one might wonder why aspergillosis is not a more common disease. Apparently normal man has developed effective defense mechanisms against these organisms. Consequently, most of the individuals who develop systemic aspergillosis have, in one way or another, a compromised immunologic responsiveness. Thus, the same type of story develops that was discussed in relationship to systemic candidiasis.

Tissue Form and Histopathology

In tissue, the PAS stain is recommended for visualizing the fungus. When any of the *Aspergillus* species invade internal organs they are characterized by the following features:
1. All form hyaline (nondematiaceous), septate hyphae.
2. All of these organisms produce dichotomously branched hyphae.
3. Under no conditions does one observe yeast cells.
4. In rare instances, in alveoli, one may observe the spore bearing heads of an *Aspergillus* species.

To see the aforementioned structures in pathology slides is an almost certain diagnosis of aspergillosis. It is possible to mistake this disease for candidiasis in tissue sections of internal organs. Strangely, under certain circumstances, *Candida* species produce hyphae that look remarkably similar to those produced by the *Aspergillus* species.

Direct Microscopic Observation

Sputum or any type of tissue should be placed on a microscope slide with 1–2 drops of 10–20% KOH. If the material is tissue, it may be necessary to tease it apart. Add a microscope coverslip and press down gently. Microscopically, with all *Aspergillus* species, one sees hyaline, dichotomously branched, septate hyphae. Occasionally in sputum, in cases of pulmonary aspergillosis, one may also see very small, rough-walled spores (3–4 microns in diameter).

Culture

All of the *Aspergillus* species grow very well on Sabouraud's medium incubated at either room temperature or 35–37 C. All *Aspergillus* species are monomorphic. Some of the species, and even some strains of certain species, grow better upon initial isolation at 35–37 C, rather than at room temperature.

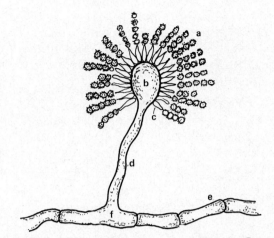

Fig 6–3.—Typical *Aspergillus* species cultured on Sabouraud's agar at either room temperature or 35–37 C. *A,* conidia (3–6 microns). *B,* vesicle. *C,* sterigma (phialide). *D,* conidiophore. *E,* septate hypha. *F,* foot cell.

For this reason I recommend that both incubation temperatures be used for initial isolation purposes.

One feature of *A. fumigatus* is often useful; it will grow at 45 C.

Because there are so many species of *Aspergillus*, the gross morphology of colonies is highly varied. Some may be black; others are green, yellow, orange or white. As this becomes a rather complex taxonomic problem, it is suggested that suspicious cultures be taken (or sent) to a mycologist for identification. The slides and Figure 6–3 suggest a preliminary idea of the microscopic morphology of *Aspergillus* species.

Aspergillus fumigatus (the most common cause of disseminated aspergillosis) produces a light green colony after 3–4 days' incubation. As the colony matures, it becomes a darker green and, eventually, after 1–2 weeks' incubation, may appear to be almost blue in color. It is not uncommon for the center portion of the colony to become a flat white color.

Other Laboratory Tests

Few other laboratory tests exist, although various serologic procedures are being experimented with. It is hoped that such tests will prove valuable enough to be released in the near future.

Therapy

The prognosis for pulmonary and disseminated aspergillosis is grave. Fungus balls may be removed surgically. Amphotericin B is usually used in cases of disseminated aspergillosis; however, the results are variable.

PHYCOMYCOSIS (ZYGOMYCOSIS)

Synonyms

Mucormycosis (an old term which should be discarded).

Definition

Phycomycosis is a systemic disease caused by a number of closely related fungi belonging to the class of fungi known as Phycomycetes. The disease may involve almost any internal organ; however, the etiologic agents seem to have a predilection for blood vessels. In some parts of the world phycomycosis may be seen as a chronic infection of subcutaneous tissue.

Etiology

Originally, all the etiologic agents of this disease were believed to belong to the order Mucorales. For this reason the term mucormycosis was developed. Since that time it has been discovered that species belonging to the following genera can also cause this disease: *Absidia, Basidiobolus, Conidiobolus, Rhizopus*. Because all of these genera belong to the class of fungi known as Phycomycetes, it was commonly accepted that the disease should be called phycomycosis. Now, however, the class Phycomycetes has been discarded, and all of the etiologic agents of this disease belong in the class Zygomycetes.

Epidemiology

Organisms belonging in the class Zygomycetes are as ubiquitous as the *Aspergillus* species. These organisms are found in soil, on all types of plant parts, including fruits, and are commonly isolated from the air any place in the world. This means that man is constantly in contact with spores of organisms belonging in the class Zygomycetes.

Predilections

As with candidiasis and aspergillosis, the systemic form of phycomycosis is most commonly found in patients who are, in one manner or another, debilitated. This disease has a distinct predilection for patients with uncontrolled diabetes mellitus, leukemia or lymphomas and for patients on prolonged therapy with antibacterial antibiotics, steroids and anticancer drugs. In such patients, the disease may spread with frightening speed, frequently resulting in death.

Tissue Form and Histopathology

To visualize these organisms in tissue, use either the PAS or methenamine silver (GMS) stains. The organisms produce very large (10–12 microns in diameter) coenocytic hyphae. Note that no yeast cells are seen as in candidiasis. These organisms differ from *Aspergillus* species in that the branching is *not* dichotomous and the hyphae lack septa. The hallmark of these organisms in tissue is the large, hyaline, coenocytic hyphae.

Direct Microscopic Examination

Any potentially infected tissue, including sputum, may be examined in KOH preparations. In such preparations, look for the relatively large, hyaline, coenocytic hyphae.

Culture

All Phycomycetes (or Zygomycetes) grow well on Sabouraud's medium. Most textbooks suggest that room temperature incubation is adequate. However, in many instances it is difficult to grow these fungi at room temperature. When incubation is at 35–37 C, many of the organisms grow more rapidly. In culture, all of the organisms grow very rapidly. After 2–3 days' incubation, masses of aerial hyphae are produced, which may fill up the entire Petri dish. The hyphae are so aerial that they may even reach up and touch the lip of the Petri dish. Most of the organisms produce gray mycelium. After 3–5 days'

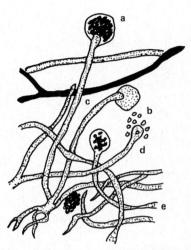

Fig 6–4.—A typical Phycomycete seen microscopically. *A*, sporangium. *B*, sporangiospores. *C*, sporangiophore. *D*, columella. *E*, coenocytic hypha.

incubation, they form spores (which are borne inside sporangia). The sporangia are jet black and are seen as minute dark specks on the aerial hyphae.

Because there is such a large number of organisms, a professional mycologist should examine cultures for further identification. Figure 6–4 is a diagrammatic representation of how members of the genus *Rhizopus* appear microscopically.

Other Laboratory Tests

Unfortunately, no other tests are currently available to aid in the diagnosis of phycomycosis.

Therapy

Very little therapy is available for the treatment of phycomycosis. If the patient has uncontrolled diabetes, it is helpful if the diabetic state can be brought into proper regulation. For patients with various types of cancer, most physicians recommend that the use of the anticancer drugs, steroids and antibacterial antibiotics be suspended. In some instances, successes have been reported with amphotericin B.

Slides

Slide 6–1.—This is a case of candidiasis of the tongue, or thrush. The tongue is covered with numerous white patches. These are microcolonies of *Candida albicans*. Underneath these yeast colonies the tongue is a bright, fiery red. Usually topical application of nystatin corrects this condition if there is no involvement of other body areas.

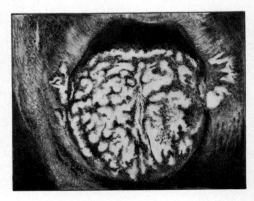

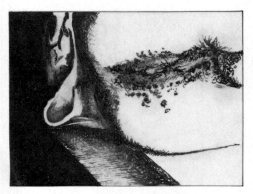

Slide 6–2.—This is a case of anal candidiasis which developed following steroid therapy.

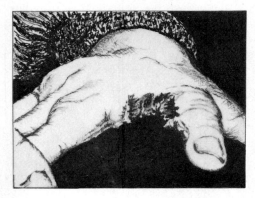

Slide 6–3.—Note the infected area between the fingers. The etiologic agent of this infection is *Candida albicans.* The patient reported that it took several months before the disease progressed to this state. In such instances, fingernails may or may not become involved.

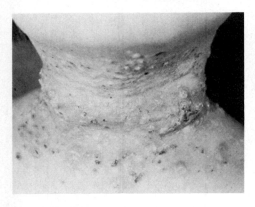

Slide 6–4.—Direct examination (KOH preparation) of infected skin indicated the presence of large numbers of a yeast. Clinical material was streaked onto Sabouraud's agar. After 2 days' incubation at room temperature all plates were covered with white yeast colonies. Further tests indicated that the organism was *Candida albicans,* leading to the diagnosis of candidiasis.

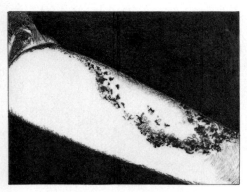

Slide 6–5.—This is a case of candidiasis on the forearm. If one were to remove skin from the periphery of the larger lesion and examine it in a KOH preparation, numerous yeast cells and occasional pseudo-hyphae would be seen.

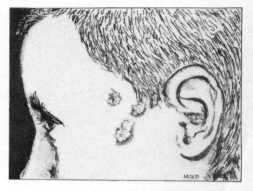

Slide 6—6.—This slide shows how candidiasis can mimic ringworm infections of the scalp.

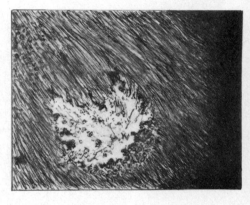

Slide 6—7.—This is a higher magnification of a scalp with candidiasis. Note how closely these lesions simulate a dermatophytic infection.

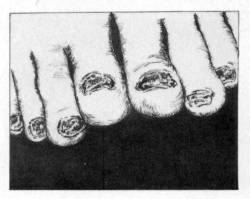

Slide 6—8.—This is a case of onychia caused by a *Candida* species. These nails have been infected for several years, and the chances of a cure are remote.

Slide 6—9.—This is a case of onychia, involving the toenails, that was caused by *Candida albicans*. Again note how this case resembles a *Trichophyton rubrum* infection of toenails.

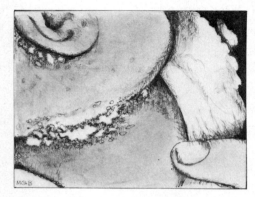

Slide 6–10.—The neck area has numerous white patches. These patches are a pure culture of *Candida albicans*.

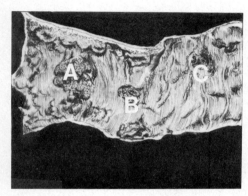

Slide 6–11.—This is a section of ileum removed from a fatal case of candidiasis. Note the numerous eruptions (A,B,C).

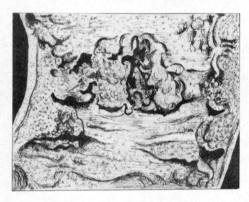

Slide 6–12.—This is from the same case of candidiasis seen in Slide 6–11 but is a higher magnification which shows the extent of destruction caused by *Candida albicans*.

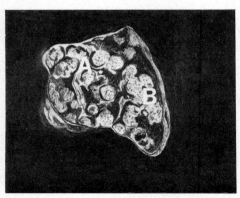

Slide 6–13.—This is a piece of kidney removed from an 8-year-old female leukemic who died of disseminated candidiasis. All of the white nodular areas on this kidney (A,B) represent areas infected with *Candida albicans*.

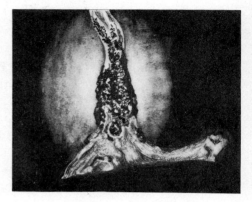

Slide 6–14.—This is the esophagus from the same patient seen in Slide 6–13. When candidiasis is disseminated, it usually is seen in the esophagus.

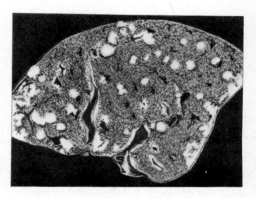

Slide 6–15.—This is the liver from a patient who had leukemia but died of disseminated candidiasis and aspergillosis. The numerous white patches are *Candida* colonies. The portion of the organ which is slightly darkened is the area of *Aspergillus* invasion.

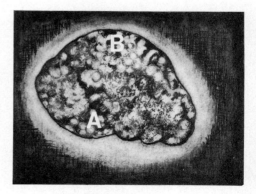

Slide 6–16.—This is another example of an organ extensively invaded with a *Candida* species. All of the white nodules (A,B) on this organ are the fungus.

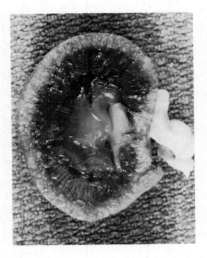

Slide 6–17.—This is a cross-sectioned kidney from a rabbit that was inoculated with *Candida albicans* 3 days previously. Observe the petechial *Candida* lesions in the cortex (outer region).

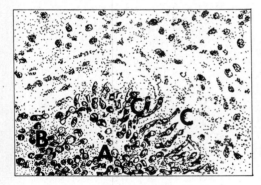

Slide 6–18.—This is a good example of how *Candida* species appear in stained sections. The fungus in this particular slide was stained by the tissue gram method (Brown and Brenn), the fungus being all of the darkly stained mass (A). Careful observation shows that in the center of the fungus colony are several yeast cells (B). On the outside of the colony the fungus seems to be growing in hyphal forms (C).

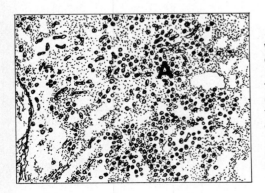

Slide 6–19.—This is a section of tissue which has been invaded by *Candida albicans*. The stain used in this preparation is methenamine silver (GMS). All of the fungal cells have taken up the silver stain (A), and they are the black structures throughout the entire slide. At this level of magnification it is difficult to discern much detail except that the organism is growing in both the yeast and the mycelial forms.

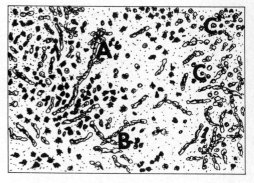

Slide 6–20. – This is from another case of systemic candidiasis. Throughout this slide are numerous hyphal strands (A,B) of *Candida albicans* which stain pink. In this particular slide it is easy to see the hyphae, but one must look carefully, especially at one side of the slide (C), in order to see the yeast cells.

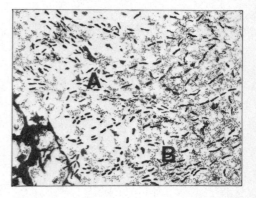

Slide 6–21. – This is a stained, frozen section done at autopsy. The diagnosis was candidiasis. Throughout the slide hyphal elements and yeast cells (A,B) can be seen.

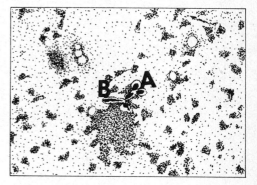

Slide 6–22. – This is how *Candida* species appear in either smears of biopsy material or sputum stained with the gram method. In the center of the slide are 4 yeast cells (A). One of them appears to be producing a pseudo-hypha (B). In some cases it is difficult to find these structures; it may be necessary to examine many microscopic fields.

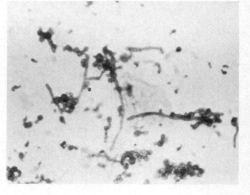

Slide 6–23. – This is a KOH preparation of freshly collected sputum. (For photographic purposes, some blue dye was added.) Note the abundance of yeast cells and pseudo-hyphae. The presence of pseudo-hyphae in freshly collected sputum should lead to the suspicion of pulmonary involvement by a *Candida* species.

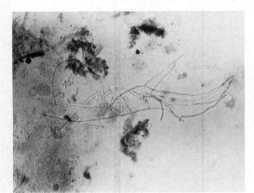

Slide 6–24.—This is another KOH preparation of freshly collected sputum (with some blue dye added). Note the abundance of long strands of pseudo-hyphae.

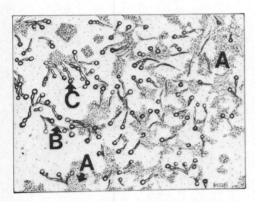

Slide 6–25.—One of the identification methods for *Candida albicans* is to observe the microscopic morphology of the organism after it has been incubated for 24–72 hours on chlamydospore or corn-meal agar. This is how *Candida albicans* looks when grown under these conditions. Because this is *Candida albicans,* one can observe 3 elements in the slide; (1) numerous yeast cells throughout the field (A), (2) occasional hyphal elements (psuedo-hyphae scattered throughout the entire field) (B) and (3) spherical cells, the chlamydospores (C), which are larger than the yeast cells.

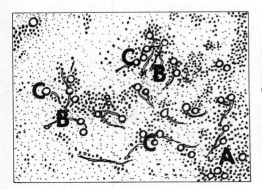

Slide 6–26.—This is another example of how *Candida albicans* appears microscopically after 24–72 hours' incubation on chlamydospore agar. As in Slide 6–25, note the abundance of yeast cells (A), occasional pseudo-hyphae (B) and the larger, spherical, dark (blue) chlamydospores (C). A combination of all 3 of these elements is needed to prove that the organism is *C. albicans.*

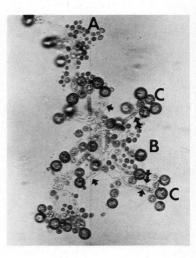

Slide 6–27. — This is a very high magnification of *C. albicans* on chlamydospore agar medium. Observe the yeast cells (A), pseudo-hyphae (B, *arrows*) and chlamydospores (C).

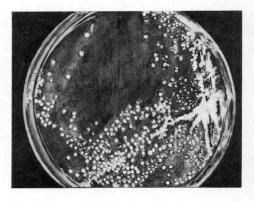

Slide 6–28. — This is how *Candida albicans* appears when cultured for 2–3 days on Sabouraud's agar incubated at either room temperature or 35–37 C. Note that it produces colonies which are very similar in morphology to many of the other yeasts and, in fact, look like many bacterial colonies to some persons.

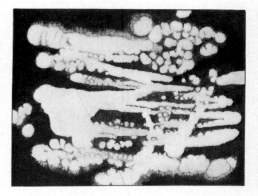

Slide 6–29. — This also is *Candida albicans,* cultured on Sabouraud's agar at either room temperature or 35–37 C for 4–5 days. Again, these are very typical appearing yeast colonies except for the "feathery" appearance around the colonies. This area is pseudo-hyphae and usually indicates a *Candida* yeast.

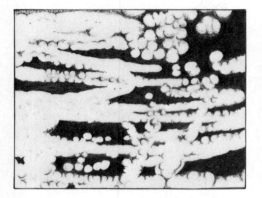

Slide 6–30.—This is a higher magnification of the colonies of *Candida albicans* shown in Slide 6–29. The colonies are said to be white to an off-white and very flat. Although some appear to have a sheen, they are usually dry-looking colonies (especially when contrasted with colonies of the encapsulated yeast, *Cryptococcus neoformans*).

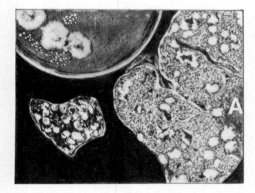

Slide 6–31.—The two organs seen in this photograph have grossly visible lesions caused by *Candida albicans*. Note an area of infarct on the liver (A); look at the curved portion of liver furthest from the Petri dish and note a darkened area (A). From this area an *Aspergillus* species was isolated. The Petri dish in this photo contains Sabouraud's medium inoculated with pieces of this liver and incubated for 3–4 days at room temperature. The 3 colonies growing on this medium are *Aspergillus fumigatus*. *A. fumigatus* colonies are usually a light green color; however, when such colonies first appear on any media they are too young to produce the green-colored spores and, therefore, the initial mass of mycelium is pure white. Thus, in this young stage, it is impossible to identify the organism. After 2–3 more days of incubation, the colonies will begin to produce spores and the characteristic green color.

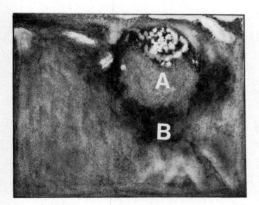

Slide 6–32.—This picture shows a pleural lesion 2–3 centimeters in diameter from a case of pulmonary aspergillosis. The red central portion (A) is composed of pulmonary parenchyma and the fungus. The dark margin (B) is the area where the blood supply has been cut off (i.e., infarcted tissue). Lesions of the pleura (surface membrane of the lung) are characteristic of *Aspergillus fumigatus* and other fungi which produce hyphae in vivo.

Slide 6–33.—This is a microscopic view of KOH prepared tissue infected with an *Aspergillus* species. Although this particular tissue is from a case of mycotic keratitis (eye infection), it is identical to infected sputum or any other type of infected tissue. Spread throughout this entire slide are masses of hyaline hyphae (A). Although not clearly evident in this photograph, the hyphae are septate and dichotomously branched. Observations of this type are important because they probably represent the first indication that the patient's disease is caused by an *Aspergillus* species.

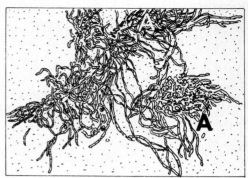

Slide 6–34.—These are hyphae of an *Aspergillus* species grown in tissue. Note that the hyphae are approximately 5–8 microns in diameter. (This fact is important when aspergillosis and phycomycosis are contrasted.) Also, in at least two places, the hyphae are branching. Because the branches divide at a 45-degree angle, this is called dichotomous branching and is characteristic of hyphae in aspergillosis. Although not seen in this picture, the hyphae of *Aspergillus* species are septate.

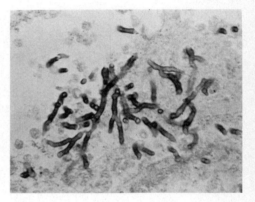

Slide 6–35.—This is another example of dichotomous branching as seen in aspergillosis.

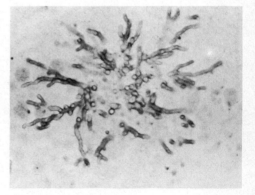

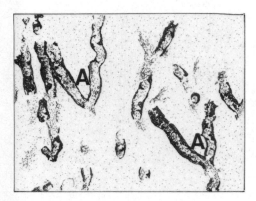

Slide 6–36.—This picture shows dichotomous branching very clearly.

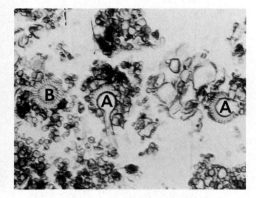

Slide 6–37.—Another tissue section of aspergillosis.

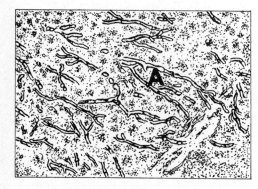

Slide 6–38.—Sometimes in air spaces in the lungs we can actually see the spore heads of an *Aspergillus* species. In this section 2 such heads are lying on the side (A,A), and 1 head is seen from the top (B). These heads (conidiophores) are the structures which give rise to the spores; they are commonly seen in cultures of *Aspergillus* species.

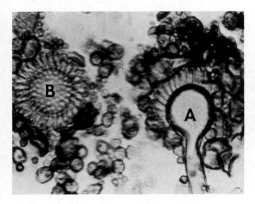

Slide 6–39.—This is a higher magnification of the conidiophores of an *Aspergillus* species as seen growing in human tissue. One conidiophore (A) is on the side and the other (B) is seen from a top view.

Slide 6–40.—This is a photomicrograph of an *Aspergillus* species grown on Sabouraud's medium at either room temperature or 35–37 C. Note the enlarged cell at the base of the conidiophore (A). This cell (B), commonly referred to as a "foot cell," is a characteristic of all *Aspergillus* species. At the upper portion of the conidiophore is a swollen head (C), referred to as a vesicle. On the vesicle is either a single row or multiple rows of sterigma (D) on which the numerous, long, slender chains of *Aspergillus* spores are borne. This is a very representative picture of the spore-bearing structure of an *Aspergillus* species.

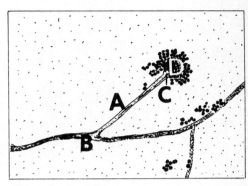

To specifically identify *Apergillus fumigatus* one must observe the color of the colony and, more important, several very fine microscopic morphological points. Here identification becomes complex; therefore, for species identification, consult a mycologist. To further illustrate this point, just a few of the taxonomic features of *Aspergillus fumigatus* will be briefly mentioned: "conidiophores short, usually densely crowded, up to 300 microns (occasionally 500 microns), two to eight microns in diameter, arising directly from submerged hyphae or as branches from aerial hyphae, septate or nonseptate, gradually enlarged, upward, with apical vesicles up to 20 to 30 microns in diameter, fertile usually only on the upper half, bearing phialides in one series, usually six to eight by two to three microns, crowded, closely packed, with axis roughly parallel to axis of the stalk. Chains of conidia form solid columns up to 400 × 50 microns. Conidia dark green in mass, globose 2–3.5 microns, mostly 2.5–3.0 microns."*

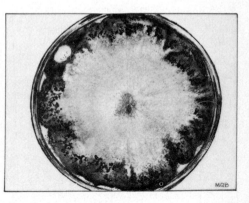

Slide 6–41.—This is a pure culture of *A. fumigatus* grown on Sabouraud's medium at either room temperature or 35 to 37 C for 2 to 3 weeks. The characteristic color of this colony is a pastel green, which darkens as the colony matures. It is not unusual for the central portion of the colony to lack color.

---

*Gilman, J. C.: *A Manual of Soil Fungi* (Ames: Iowa State University Press, 1957), pp. 219–220.

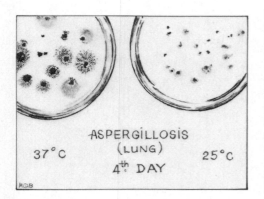

Slide 6–42.—This is a rather interesting photograph from which a lesson can be learned. Recently we saw a case of pulmonary aspergillosis and, as usual, inoculated samples of tissue on Sabouraud's agar and incubated them at room temperature and 37 C. Note that the colonies of the 37 C plate grew out more rapidly than those colonies incubated at room temperature. In fact, the green color of the colonies that were incubated at 37 C is beginning to be visible. This picture clearly demonstrates that certain of the opportunistic pathogens may grow better when incubated at the elevated temperature.

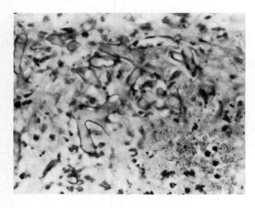

Slide 6–43.—In contrast to aspergillosis, the hyphae seen in tissue with phycomycosis are much larger (usually 10–15 microns in diameter) and are not septate, i.e., are coenocytic. This slide shows the characteristic hyphae seen in phycomycosis.

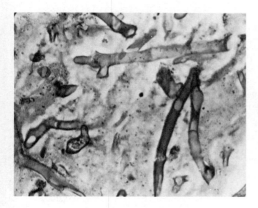

Slide 6–44.—This is another example of hyphae seen in phycomycosis.

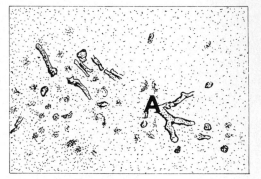

Slide 6–45.—More phycomycosis hyphae (A).

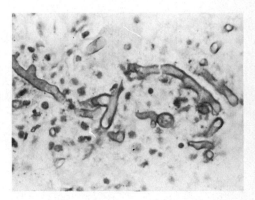

Slide 6–46.—Note that all these hyphae are coenocytic: phycomycosis.

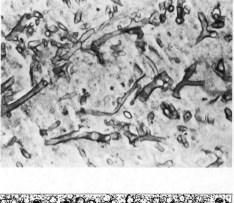

Slide 6–47.—All of these hyphal elements are 10–15 microns in diameter and are coenocytic. Occasionally one might think that a septum is present; usually this is an area where the hyphae have bent, thus creating the appearance of a crosswall.

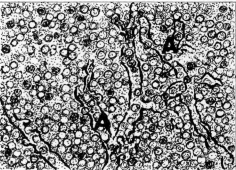

Slide 6–48.—This is the microscopic appearance of the coenocytic hyphae (A) in a KOH preparation of sputum from a patient with phycomycosis. Because the hyphae are hyaline, they may be difficult to discern.

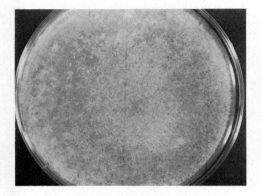

Slide 6–49.—This is a young culture of a *Rhizopus* or *Mucor* species. Note the rapid spread of the colony and the large number of aerial hyphae. (In fact, the hyphae are touching the inside of the lid of the Petri dish.) The small black dots are sporangia. In 1–2 days more the colony would be a darker gray or brown color and completely fill up the Petri dish.

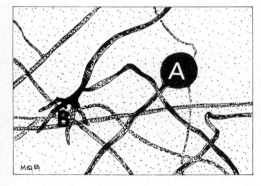

Slide 6–50.—This is a photomicrograph of a *Rhizopus* species grown on Sabouraud's medium and incubated at either room temperature or 35 to 37 C. The darkly stained, spherical structure is the sporangium (A). As the sporangium matures further, it will contain numerous sporangiospores. Note where the sporangiophore connects with the hypha; these finger-like structures are called rhizoids (B) and are characteristic for the genus *Rhizopus* (see Fig 6–4).

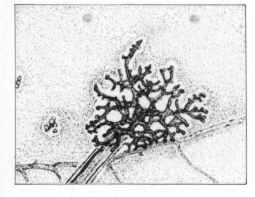

Slide 6–51.—This is a high magnification photomicrograph of the characteristic rhizoids of the genus *Rhizopus*.

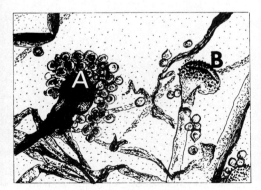

Slide 6–52.—This is another photomicrograph of a *Rhizopus* species; however, this is from a much older culture. The sporangia have matured and broken open. On one of the spore heads (A) are numerous spores ready to be released. The other spore head (B) is completely devoid of spores. This is a rather characteristic picture for an older culture of either *Rhizopus* or *Mucor*. In addition to these structures one should determine if the hyphae are coenocytic and whether rhizoids are present.

As with the *Aspergillus* species, members of the class Phycomycetes (or Zygomycetes) are rather difficult to identify to the species level, and the culture should be shown to a mycologist.

For present purposes, as far as phycomycosis is concerned, it is sufficient to observe relatively large, nondematiaceous, coenocytic, nondichotomously branched hyphae in vivo and an extremely fluffy culture. This does not mean that complete identification of an etiologic agent is unimportant, but the therapy is the same for this disease regardless of the specific etiologic agent involved. Therefore, for the patient's sake, first determine whether the disease is phycomycosis, institute therapy and then seek taxonomic assistance from a mycologist.

SELF-EVALUATION QUESTIONS
(Answers at end of questions)

Select the ONE best answer for each question:

1. In vivo, *Candida albicans* produces
   a. _____ yeast cells
   b. _____ hyphae
   c. _____ yeast cells and hyphae
   d. _____ yeast cells, hyphae and chlamydospores
2. Etiologic agents of phycomycosis (or zygomycosis) include members of the following genera:
   a. _____ *Rhizopus*
   b. _____ *Mucor*
   c. _____ *Absidia*
   d. _____ all of the above
3. Which one of the following diseases is endogenous in origin?
   a. _____ aspergillosis
   b. _____ candidiasis
   c. _____ phycomycosis
   d. _____ all of the above
4. The outstanding characteristics of *Aspergillus* species growing in tissue are:
   a. _____ hyaline, septate, dichotomously branched hyphae
   b. _____ pseudo-hyphae
   c. _____ coenocytic hyphae
   d. _____ pseudo-hyphae and chlamydospores
5. The drug of choice for dermal, oral and vaginal candidiasis is
   a. _____ griseofulvin
   b. _____ amphotericin B
   c. _____ gentian violet
   d. _____ nystatin
6. Occasionally, in alveoli, one will see the spore heads of
   a. _____ *Rhizopus* species
   b. _____ *Mucor* species
   c. _____ *Aspergillus* species
   d. _____ *Candida* species

7. *Candida albicans* can be identified on chlamydospore or cornmeal agar when one observes
   a. _____ pseudo-hyphae
   b. _____ yeast cells
   c. _____ chlamydospores
   d. _____ all of the above
8. Which of the following diseases are produced by several organisms?
   a. _____ candidiasis
   b. _____ phycomycosis (zygomycosis)
   c. _____ aspergillosis
   d. _____ all of the above
9. Assimilation tests are necessary to identify
   a. _____ *Candida* species
   b. _____ *Aspergillus* species
   c. _____ *Mucor* species
   d. _____ *Rhizopus* species
10. Considering what you now know about aspergillosis, what is the most probable portal of entry?
    a. _____ puncture wound
    b. _____ blood
    c. _____ lungs
    d. _____ gastrointestinal tract

Complete the following sentences by filling in the blanks:

11. In tissue, all *Candida* species form _____ and _____.
12. The colony of *Aspergillus fumigatus* is a _____ color.
13. The hyphae of all Phycomycetes (or zygomycetes) are _____.
14. The recommended medium for the primary isolation of *Candida albicans* is _____.
15. A "fungus ball" may be formed by _____ species.
16. An older (obsolete) name for phycomycosis (or zygomycosis) is _____.
17. Three genera of fungi which may cause phycomycosis (or zygomycosis) are _____, _____ and _____.
18. The most common cause of aspergillosis is _____.
19. One major problem with nystatin is that it cannot be used _____.
20. The most common cause of candidiasis is *Candida* _____.

Answers to questions 1–20.

1. c	11. yeast, pseudo-hyphae
2. d	12. green
3. b	13. coenocytic (and hyaline)
4. a	14. Sabouraud's
5. d	15. *Aspergillus*
6. c	16. mucormycosis
7. d	17. *Rhizopus, Mucor, Absidia*
8. d	18. *A. fumigatus*
9. a	19. systemically
10. c	20. *albicans*

7 / Central Nervous System Mycoses

SEVERAL FUNGUS DISEASES show a predilection for the central nervous system (CNS). Such infections may be classified in the following categories.

CHRONIC MENINGITIS.—Infections of this type may be "silent," which means that they may have existed for extended periods of time with few noticeable clinical symptoms. On the other hand, some patients report headache, dizziness, nausea, vomiting and a stiff neck. Although these are symptoms of several of the mycoses involving the brain, they also may be symptoms of many nonmycotic CNS disorders. The fungus diseases that most frequently cause chronic meningitis are cryptococcosis, coccidioidomycosis and histoplasmosis.

CEREBRAL ABSCESSES.—These are intracerebral expanding masses. The symptoms for this type of disorder depend on the location of the lesion. Nocardiosis is often implicated in cerebral abscesses; occasionally candidiasis and dematiaceous infectious (cladosporiosis) are involved.

CEREBRAL INFARCTS.—Mycotic infarcts are usually caused by fungi which form hyphae in vivo. In these instances, rapidly progressive focal lesions develop, leading to cerebral vascular accident (CVA) symptoms. The most commonly implicated mycoses causing infarcts are phycomycosis (zygomycosis) and aspergillosis.

Because many of the diseases just mentioned have been discussed in previous chapters, only a brief review of some of their important features will be given here.

COCCIDIOIDOMYCOSIS

For coccidioidomycosis, serologic information is of great value diagnostically, prognostically and therapeutically. When clinical material is available, it should be examined in KOH preparations and stained slides for the presence of spherules and endospores. Some of this material may be cultured on Sabouraud's agar (but, remember, the etiologic agent is a laboratory hazard) incubated at room temperature. After 3 weeks' incubation the organism, *Coccidioides immitis*, appears as a white, fluffy colony and, microscopically, is characterized by the formation of arthrospores.

CANDIDIASIS

Fortunately, candidiasis rarely causes brain disease. When reported, this disease is usually found in patients with diabetes, those receiving extended antibiotic or steroid therapy, those who have had recent brain surgery or those with indwelling catheters for extended time periods.

In direct examination of histopathological preparations, one looks for the presence of pseudo-hyphae and yeast cells. Material should be cultured on Sabouraud's agar and incubated at room temperature and at 35–37 C. White yeast colonies appear after 2–3 days' incubation. Subculture onto an identification medium such as chlamydospore or cornmeal agar. After 24–72 hours of incubation, *Candida albicans* forms yeast cells, pseudo-hyphae and chlamydospores.

ASPERGILLOSIS

Aspergillosis is usually a fatal disease when there is brain involvement. Diagnosis is extremely difficult because no really good serologic tools are commercially available. In tissue, the etiologic agents are characterized by the formation of septate, dichotomously branched hyphae. *Aspergillus* species may be cultured at either room temperature or 35–37 C on Sabouraud's medium. All of the etiologic agents are monomorphic. Species identification is difficult and is usually made by a mycologist.

DEMATIACEOUS INFECTIONS

Dematiacious fungi are any fungi whose hyphae are brown. In recent years many reports have appeared concerning subcutaneous and brain abscesses caused by various types of dematiacious fungi. Because the genus *Cladosporium* has frequently been implicated, some authors call this disease "cladosporiosis." Others prefer "phaeohyphomycosis," or a form of chromomycosis.

In tissue, these fungi produce brown septate hyphae which occasionally contain thick-walled chlamydospores. No yeast cells, granules or fission (sclerotic) bodies are formed; thus, this disease is different from chromomycosis and mycetoma. Unfortunately, most brain abscesses caused by dematiacious fungi are diagnosed at autopsy. No serologic tools are available for diagnostic purposes. All of the etiologic agents grow on Sabouraud's medium incubated at room temperature. Some of them grow at 35–37 C or even higher. Most of the colonies are brown to black. A mycologist should identify specific genera.

HISTOPLASMOSIS

In cases of histoplasmosis, serologic information can be of great value diagnostically, prognostically and therapeutically. When clinical material is available, it should be examined with Wright's or Giemsa stained smears and PAS stained slides. In tissue, *Histoplasma capsulatum* grows as a very small intracellular yeast.

Culture clinical material on Sabouraud's medium incubated at room temperature and on brain-heart infusion agar incubated at 35–37 C. At room temperature the colony usually is a fluffy white color and microscopically has the characteristic tuberculated macroaleuriospores and the infectious microaleuriospores. Grown at 35–37 C, the fungus produces a white to light brown yeast colony. Microscopically, one observes numerous very small yeast cells and no hyphae. *H. capsulatum* is a true dimorphic fungus.

NOCARDIOSIS

Nocardiosis frequently produces pyogenic lesions of the brain and meninges. No serological tools are available for diagnostic purposes. As the etiologic agents of this disease are "higher bacteria," they form very fine, delicately branched, gram-positive and partially acid-fast filaments, both in tissue and in laboratory culture. When sectioned tissue preparations are made, the tissue gram stain (Brown and Brenn) and acid-fast stains are recommended. These organisms grow well on Sabouraud's medium incubated at either room temperature or 35–37 C. At either temperature, cultures take 1–3 weeks to develop. The colonies are very compact, wrinkled and not fluffy. They vary from chalky in appearance to yellow to orange to brown. Microscopically, numerous very fine, delicately branched filaments can be observed.

PHYCOMYCOSIS (OR ZYGOMYCOSIS)

Phycomycosis includes etiologic agents belonging to the class Phycomycetes (Zygomycetes). Example genera are *Absidia, Mucor* and *Rhizopus*. Often these organisms invade the brain through the nasal pharynx and grow in and around the vessels. By growing in vessels they cause infarcts. Diagnosis of phycomycosis is very difficult and is usually made at autopsy. No diagnostic serologic tools are available.

In either direct examination preparations or in tissue slides, these organisms produce broad, coenocytic hyphae. In PAS stained preparations, the hyphae stain pink. All of these organisms are monomorphic, i.e., they grow the same way on Sabouraud's agar at either room temperature or 35–37 C. Usually the colonies develop relatively rapidly and produce considerable amounts of gray to black aerial hyphae which, after 5–6 days' incubation, may actually fill up a Petri dish. A mycologist should identify specific genera.

In the remainder of this chapter I shall discuss cryptococcosis as a general example of a CNS mycosis.

CRYPTOCOCCOSIS

Synonyms

Torulosis, European blastomycosis.

Definition

Cryptococcosis is an acute or chronic, and pulmonary, systemic or meningeal mycosis. The pulmonary form may be transitory and may pass unrecognized. Although various organs may become involved, subacute or chronic meningitis is the most familiar form.

Etiology

Although there are several species belonging to the genus *Cryptococcus*, the only one that causes a disease in man is *C. neoformans*. The organism is well named because the prefix "crypto" is Greek for "hidden." In microbiological terms this means that the organism is surrounded by a capsule. *C. neoformans* is the only encapsulated yeast which is pathogenic to man. The perfect (sexual) phase of this organism has been placed in the genus *Filobasidiella*.

Epidemiology

C. neoformans is found worldwide growing in soils, especially those containing pigeon feces. In these conditions the organism is saprophytic. It may maintain a saprophytic existence for years. After being disseminated by wind currents, it supposedly enters the human lung and induces a disease state.

Although the disease cryptococcosis was first described in the late 1800s, until recently it was considered to be an extremely rare disease. Now, with increasing frequency, cases are being reported all over the world. We still do not know how common this disease may be; however, one authority speculated that each year in New York City alone there are between 5,000 and 15,000 clinical to subclinical cases of cryptococcosis.

Predilections

As far as can be determined, many of the patients having cryptococcosis are devoid of obvious predisposing factors. On the other hand, it is not uncommon to find this disease in patients with Hodgkin's disease, lymphoma or tuberculosis. Some persons believe that certain forms of surgery (especially those involving organ transplants) and prolonged therapy with steroids predispose one to cryptococcosis.

Direct Microscopic Examination

As this disease is most frequently diagnosed in the meningeal form, spinal fluid is the material commonly used for direct examination and culture purposes. If lung involvement is suspected, one may use sputum or biopsy material.

Place material to be examined directly on a microscope slide and add 1–2 drops of slightly diluted India ink (in some parts of the world called "China" ink). Place a coverslip on this preparation and press down gently. Microscopically, this organism is seen as yeast cells, 8–12 microns in diameter, which are usually surrounded by huge, clear capsules that may be twice the diameter of the yeast cells.

Tissue Form and Histopathology

If tissue is available for sectioning, it should be stained with either PAS or mucicarmine. Look for encapsulated yeast cells.

Culture

Since *C. neoformans* is monomorphic, it grows as a yeast on Sabouraud's medium at either room temperature or 35–37 C. The colonies develop after 1–3 weeks' incubation as shiny, slimy, light tan yeast colonies. These colonies may be so slimy that if the Petri dish or test tube is incubated on a slant, the colony flows toward the bottom. Microscopically, in India ink preparations, one looks for encapsulated yeast cells. This organism rarely forms hyphae, almost always produces a capsule and is urease positive.

Other Laboratory Tests

Laboratories have begun to use serologic tests as a diagnostic aid for cryptococcosis. One of these tests (latex agglutination) is commercially available in some parts of the world; many persons are not yet certain that it is of diagnostic and prognostic value.

Following either intraperitoneal or intracerebral inoculation of *C. neoformans* into mice, fatal cryptococcosis results.

Therapy

If allowed to run its course, cryptococcal meningitis is usually fatal. In recent years, amphotericin B has been used successfully in many cases *if* a diagnosis can be reached at a relatively early stage in the development of the disease. Some recent reports indicate that 5-fluorocytosine has been used with some success. Isolated cryptococcomas in the lung may be removed surgically. This type of treatment has been successful in many instances, especially when the patient is given concurrent and follow-up therapy with amphotericin B.

OPTIONAL SECTION (for advanced students)

The remainder of this chapter departs from the usual format. Previous chapters have presented material in a straightforward, organized fashion. This was done with the hope that such presentations would make the learning process simpler for those beginning to study the important fungal pathogens. However, presenting material in such a fashion may leave the impression that medical mycology is dull, unimaginative and unchallenging. Such is not the case. The fungi, as human pathogens, should represent a great challenge to the medical researcher. Our knowledge in many areas of mycology is extremely limited; thus there is a great need for research. For these reasons, cryptococcosis will be discussed from an experimental point of view. Some questions will be presented that we began to ask in our research laboratories some 15 years ago. Think about these questions; try to decide how to approach the problem experimentally. Then some of our thinking on the subject, our approach to the problems, some of our experimental models, the data that we obtained from these experiments and some of the current thinking on the subject of the pathogenesis of cryptococcosis will be presented. This approach may show that medical mycology can be an exciting and challenging field and what type of research can be done in it.

The first question is: "Why doesn't everyone in the world contract cryptococcosis?" The organism and the disease are found worldwide. The organism grows readily in soil containing pigeon feces, and pigeons are found everywhere. This means that it is probably not uncommon for man to be exposed to *Cryptococcus neoformans*. As not all of us come down with cryptococcosis, there must be some rather effective body defense mechanisms at work against the organism. If one decides to look at this aspect, what body defenses should be selected for initial investigation? Although there are many that could be investigated, we decided initially to look at the process of phagocytosis. This is the process in which the white blood cells (leukocytes) engulf and, in most cases, kill foreign microbes which enter the body. Phagocytosis and many related events are referred to as cellular immunity, and this aspect of human defense mechanisms is considered to be particularly important in the mycoses.

The first experiment we decided on was to see how well peripheral human leukocytes engulfed cells of *C. neoformans*. Human blood was expressed onto a microscope slide. After a brief incubation period the film of red blood cells

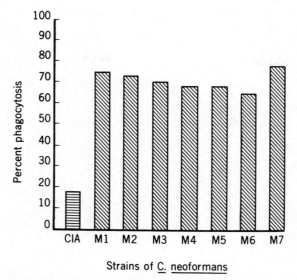

Fig 7–1.— A comparison of phagocytosis between an encapsulated *C. neoformans* (CIA) and nonencapsulated mutants (M1 – M7).

was removed, leaving a suspension of white blood cells on the slide. After adding cells of *C. neoformans*, we added a coverslip and observed the suspension microscopically. Although it was delightful to see the phagocytic cells crawling about, extending pseudopods here and there, we were disappointed because in only a few instances did we observe the white cells engulfing yeast cells. Eventually, we devised a quantitative method for determining percent phagocytosis (the number of white blood cells which engulfed cells of *C. neoformans*), and, in all instances, less than 20% of the white blood cells engulfed cells of *C. neoformans*. This was not only a disappointment but raised a second important question: "Why didn't human white blood cells engulf the cells of *C. neoformans?*" Look at a picture of *C. neoformans* (e.g., Slide 7 – 15) to see whether there is anything that might be inhibiting the phagocytic process. We hypothesized that perhaps the huge capsule which completely surrounds the cell might interfere with the phagocytic process. If this were true, the percent phagocytosis would be much higher if the capsule were absent. To investigate this premise, we set out to isolate nonencapsulated mutants of *C. neoformans*. Eventually we isolated 7 strains of nonencapsulated mutants using ultraviolet irradiation on an encapsulated strain. Again, we did the phagocytosis experiments. We were delighted to record the data presented in Figure 7 – 1. To us, these data meant that the capsule must in some way be inhibiting the phagocytic process. The parent encapsulated strain (CIA) was phagocytized very poorly: however, all of the 7 nonencapsulated mutants (M1 – M7) were phagocytized at much higher rates, in fact, 3 to 4 times higher.

We then decided to pursue two lines of investigation.

First, we prepared suspensions of the parent encapsulated cells and all of the nonencapsulated mutants and injected them into mice. As one might expect, the animals injected with the parent encapsulated strain died of disseminated cryptococcosis. Much to our pleasure, few of the animals injected with nonencapsulated mutants died of cryptococcosis. This simple experiment led

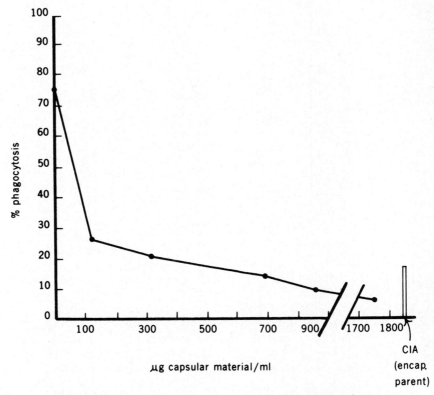

Fig 7–2. — Inhibition of in vitro phagocytosis of nonencapsulated mutants of *C. neoformans* by capsular material.

us to the conclusion that perhaps the capsule of *C. neoformans* is a virulence factor.

Second, we decided to do more quantitative experiments on the inhibition of phagocytosis by cryptococcal capsular material. To do this, we removed (with a sonic oscillator) large amounts of capsular material from the parent encapsulated strain. This material was subsequently purified and eventually was recovered as a dry, white powder. We then did another phagocytosis experiment in which we used human peripheral leukocytes and one of the nonencapsulated mutants. We set up several tubes containing this mixture. To one of these tubes nothing further was added, and to the other tubes increasing amounts of the purified capsular material were added. After a suitable incubation period we assayed for the percent phagocytosis in each of the tubes. The data we obtained from this experiment are shown in Figure 7–2. Phagocytosis in the tube which contained no capsular material was between 70% and 80%. With the addition of approximately 150 micrograms of capsular material, phagocytosis was less than 30%. As more and more capsular material was added, the percent phagocytosis decreased even further. From these data we concluded that even in microgram amounts the capsule of *C. neoformans* inhibited phagocytosis.

All of this is perhaps interesting, but what does it have to do with body defense mechanisms against this pathogen? After all, who ever heard of

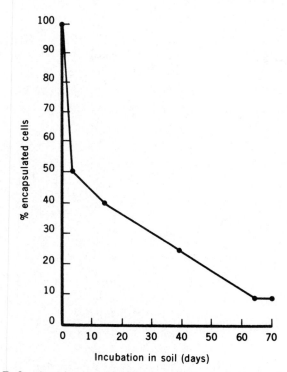

Fig 7–3. — Incubation of 8 strains of *C. neoformans* in soil.

nonencapsulated mutants of *C. neoformans* outside of the laboratory experiments just described? These are good questions, and they concerned us for some time. However, we then asked: What do we know about the infectious particle of *C. neoformans?* Do we know that it is always encapsulated? No, we do not. This led us into a series of experiments in which we took heavily encapsulated cells of *C. neoformans* and inoculated them into soil. After varying incubation periods we examined the cells microscopically and recorded the size of the cell and the amount of capsule present. These observations are recorded in Figure 7–3. To us, these data meant only one thing, namely, that during soil incubation of a heavily encapsulated strain of *C. neoformans* the capsule gradually disappears. Additionally, we noted that with the disappearance of the capsule the cell became smaller. Perhaps *C. neoformans* resides in soil in a form completely different from that we observe in the human host and in laboratory culture. From these data we proposed that the infectious particle of *C. neoformans* is actually a relatively small, nonencapsulated yeast cell.

What do we have so far? We have the possibility that the infectious particle of *C. neoformans* is a relatively small, nonencapsulated yeast which resides in soil. On the other hand, it appears that the capsule is a virulence factor which is a potent inhibitor of phagocytosis. Is that the complete story? What are the weak points? What experiment should now be performed to try to pull together these two seemingly isolated premises? We decided that it was important to know if the nonencapsulated infectious particles could produce capsular material in vivo and, if so, how long this process takes. Information of this

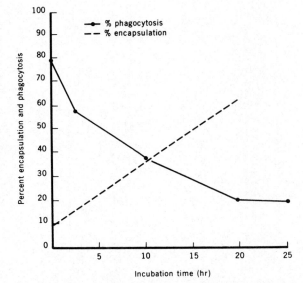

Fig 7–4. — Capsular production and phagocytosis of *C. neoformans* in human lung tissue in vitro.

type would indicate how much time the phagocytic process had to function in an effective manner before the antiphagocytic capsular material was produced in sufficient amounts to inhibit phagocytosis. Obviously we could not use the encapsulated parent cell or the nonencapsulated mutants for this type of experiment. This meant that we had to devise ways to culture encapsulated cells of *C. neoformans* in a nonencapsulated state. If this could be done, the nonencapsulated state would be, according to our theory, a simulation of the infectious particle. Eventually, we devised several methods to inhibit capsule production in vitro. Now we were ready to determine how much time was required before environmentally induced nonencapsulated cells of *C. neoformans* produced sufficient amounts of capsular material to inhibit phagocytosis. To do this experiment, we wanted to utilize to the greatest possible extent natural material and conditions. The Department of Pathology gave us several pieces of normal human lung which were obtained, just a short time before our experiment began, from a patient whose cause of death was a nonrespiratory problem. We began the experiment by incubating the environmentally induced nonencapsulated cells of *C. neoformans* in a large test tube containing small pieces of the lung tissue and saline. At varying times during the 37 C incubation, we removed portions of the fluid containing the *Cryptococcus* cells and attempted to visualize the amount of capsule on the cells. Additionally, we added the yeast cells to a typical phagocytosis experiment, as previously described, and recorded percent phagocytosis. Thus, plotted against time, we attempted to observe capsule production visually and also to record this process, using inhibition of phagocytosis as an index. The data we obtained are recorded in Figure 7–4. To us, these data meant the following:

1. At time zero phagocytosis was near 80%.
2. As incubation time increased, the nonencapsulated cells began to produce capsular material (see dotted line).

Approximately 2½ hours after the nonencapsulated cells were incubated with the lung material, these cells produced sufficient capsular material to inhibit phagocytosis by more than 20%; i.e., after 2½ hours' incubation, phagocytosis was down to 55–60%. With increased incubation time the percent phagocytosis decreased even further. After 15–20 hours' incubation, phagocytosis was approximately 25%.

From these data we concluded that only a few hours after the nonencapsulated infectious particle enters the human body, it begins to produce sufficient capsular material to inhibit phagocytosis. Thus, if phagocytosis is an effective defense mechanism against *C. neoformans,* it must function rather rapidly. Should this process be delayed in any fashion, then the organism would produce sufficient capsular material to inhibit the phagocytic process.

Now I raise the question: "What flaws can you see in this theory?" In all of the experiments described above, we have never proved that phagocytes can kill engulfed cells of *C. neoformans.* This was the next series of experiments that we attempted. Initially we experimented with human peripheral leukocytes. Much to our pleasure, we discovered that phagocytized nonencapsulated yeast cells were killed rapidly. Then, realizing that most people consider the lung to be the primary portal of entry of *C. neoformans,* we decided to repeat these experiments using lung macrophages. Despite numerous attempts and varied experimental approaches, we have never been able to demonstrate the killing of engulfed cells of *C. neoformans* in vitro by lung macrophages.

If the lung truly is the primary portal of entry, the fact that lung macrophages do not kill engulfed cells of *C. neoformans* presents a rather puzzling situation. Probably the lung macrophages are not primary killing cells. Perhaps these scavenger cells engulf cells of *C. neoformans* and then dispose of them by another mechanism or another route. For example, could the lung macrophage function by carrying the cells of *C. neoformans* into the gastrointestinal tract where they are eliminated? This could be true, and, in fact, is currently being investigated. On the other hand, perhaps the lung macrophages function by carrying the yeast cells to another site, where they are killed by other mechanisms. This method could result in the development of cryptococcomas in certain individuals. Cryptococcomas might be areas of compartmentalization where the potential pathogen is either killed or held in a state of stasis; at a later date they might function as dissemination depots.

Undoubtedly, these experiments raise many questions. On the other hand, some of the experiments help us to see a little more clearly how and why certain individuals contract cryptococcosis. In this regard, following are some thoughts about the data.

It now appears that *C. neoformans* probably resides in the soil as a relatively small nonencapsulated yeast cell. In retrospect, this seems very logical, because how can a heavily encapsulated cell that may be 15–30 microns in diameter gain entrance into the human lung? From what is known about lung anatomy and physiology, a particle of this size is too large to enter the human lung to any appreciable depth. However, a nonencapsulated infectious particle, one that is probably less than 5 microns in diameter, would have a much better chance of penetrating the lung milieu. Additionally, if the infectious particle lacks a capsule, the white blood cells in the human body could more readily engulf and kill this yeast. If peripheral leukocytes are capable of both engulfing and killing cells of *C. neoformans*, this may explain why the skin has never been considered a portal of entry for cells of *C. neoformans*.

Now what about the lung? Under normal conditions, lung macrophages will phagocytize the nonencapsulated infectious particles. Although they may not function as primary killing cells, they probably have alternative mechanisms of disposing of the potential pathogens.

How do all of these considerations relate to the fact that only certain individuals develop cryptococcosis? In this regard, following are three proposals:

1. It is conceivable that certain individuals might come in contact with massive amounts of cells of *C. neoformans* in aerosols. Perhaps these are people working in dusty areas, and the dust contains great numbers of cells of *C. neoformans*. As with all body organs and tissues, there is a level of overload. Perhaps millions of cells of *C. neoformans* entering the human body in a relatively short period of time would overload the phagocytic process to such a point that phagocytosis is transiently inhibited. Should such a situation develop and phagocytosis be inhibited for only a few hours, then the nonencapsulated cells of this organism would have sufficient time to produce enough antiphagocytic capsular material to inhibit phagocytosis further. The organism would then begin to replicate, and the ensuing progeny would produce more capsular material. This could lead to a point where the phagocytic process is overwhelmed, and an infection would then result.

2. If phagocytosis is a truly important defense mechanism against cells of *C. neoformans*, what would happen if the process were inhibited by such means as the administration of various drugs, surgery or numerous other known and unknown factors? Perhaps permanent or even transient depressions in phagocytosis are genetically controlled. Regardless of the mechanism, be it inborn or induced or an alteration in the normal physiological functionings of our body, the result would be the same. As indicated in Proposal 1, the nonencapsulated infectious particles might then have sufficient time to produce the antiphagocytic capsular material. This proposal differs from the first one in that large numbers of infectious particles would not be needed to establish an infection.

3. At one point, the establishment of cryptococcomas was mentioned. Could such structures be more common than currently suspected? Perhaps many people have inhaled cells of *C. neoformans* but, through some mechanism, the yeast cells have been sequestered and held in stasis for extended periods of time. This concept could lead one to speculate that many cases of disseminated cryptococcosis originate from latent infections, i.e., cryptococcoma-like structures. Perhaps such structures could contain viable cells of *C. neoformans* for periods of months or even years. Then at some time when the delicate balance between the host and the potential pathogen is altered to favor the pathogen, these quiescent cells of *C. neoformans* could be revitalized and begin to reproduce again and disseminate. Thus, *Cryptococcus neoformans* might really be an opportunistic fungus. As stated previously, this organism is found worldwide, which means that everyone must be exposed to it. Since not everyone contracts this disease, perhaps the susceptible indi-

vidual is one whose normal body defenses have been temporarily thrown off balance. This imbalance could create an environment which would favor the proliferation of organisms like *C. neoformans*.

Now look at this disease, or any other fungus disease, and ask some questions. This is the process which eventually provides answers, and only with knowledge of this type will better methods of controlling the insidious mycoses be found.

In this chapter, we have discussed several fungus diseases that have been presented earlier in the book. Refer to the photographs and sketches in previous chapters for the ways that these organisms look in vivo and in vitro. As dematiaceous infections and cryptococcosis have not been presented previously, pictures relating to these two diseases will be shown.

Slides

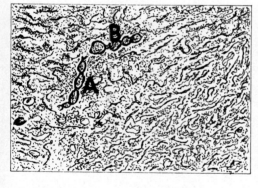

Slide 7–1. — This is a photomicrograph of material obtained from a skin abscess containing dematiacious fungal elements. It does not make any difference if the material is from a skin or a brain abscess; the fungal elements in this disease appear the same. Near the center of the slide (A,B) the hyphal elements are brown. The hyphae contain numerous somewhat rounded cells, almost as though chlamydospores are being formed.

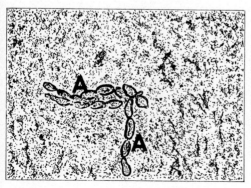

Slide 7–2. — This is another photomicrograph of a dematiacious infection. This particular preparation was made from pus taken from a brain abscess. The fungus is represented by brown hyphal elements (A) in the center of the field which have a tendency to form chlamydospores.

Slide 7–3.—As indicated above, it is not necessary to prepare stained sectioned slides from cases of dematiacious infections. In most instances, a direct examination preparation is sufficient. Perhaps for other reasons, tissue may be removed, sectioned and stained in the normal manner. If this is done, dematiacious fungi (which are normally seen as brown hyphae) take up some of the stain and in a PAS stain they appear to be a pink color. These hyphal elements (A,B) are septate, and have random branching and a tendency toward chlamydospore formation.

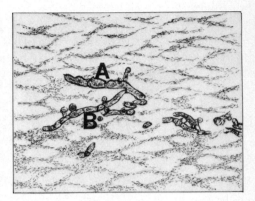

Regardless of the source or site of infection and the specific etiologic agent in dematiaceous infections, one will always see structures similar to those shown in these three slides. Along with these observations and the repeated culturing of a dematiacious fungus, one may conclude, with a high degree of certainty, that the patient has a dematiacious infection.

Slide 7–4.—Most often, cryptococcosis presents clinically as a meningitis. Because slides of meningitis patients are of little value, pictures of patients with pulmonary cryptococcosis will be shown. This particular patient supposedly had tuberculosis many years ago. After appropriate therapy she was considered cured. However, following a bump on the shoulder, she deteriorated, over a period of several months, to the state seen in this picture. Eventually it was discovered that she had pulmonary cryptococcosis.

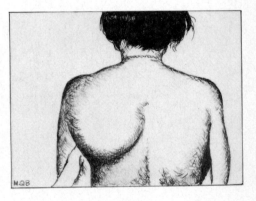

Slide 7–5.—The patient was treated surgically, with removal of the infected area and followup therapy with amphotericin B. To this date, 5–6 years later, she is apparently quite well. In this picture one can see the two ribs which were removed from her chest. Note that the upper rib (A) is almost totally destroyed and the other rib (B) has considerable erosion. Fortunately, invasion and destruction of bone tissue of the type shown in the slide are rare in patients with cryptococcosis.

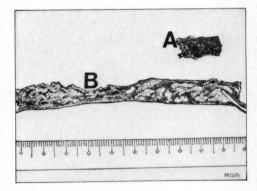

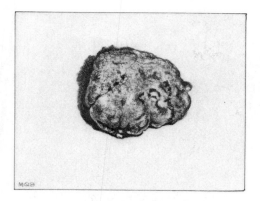

Slide 7–6.—This is a cryptococcoma removed from another patient with pulmonary cryptococcosis. Note the size and walled-off nature of this structure. After removal of the cryptococcoma, the patient was placed on extended amphotericin B therapy and recovered completely. Both of the patients just shown were from Southeast Asia, where, in my experience, a greater number of cases of *pulmonary* cryptococcosis seem to occur than are routinely seen in the Americas.

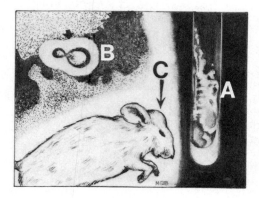

Slide 7–7.—This is a composite picture of some of the procedures we undertook to identify *Cryptococcus neoformans* removed from the patient seen in Slide 7–4. At one corner of this slide is the test tube (A) containing the slimy culture of *C. neoformans*. At the other side of the slide is an India ink preparation from this culture (B). Note the heavily encapsulated, budding yeast cells. Additionally, we inoculated some clinical material into the brains of young mice (C). Five days later these animals died. Before death, they had obvious CNS disturbances, and the cap of the skull was elevated.

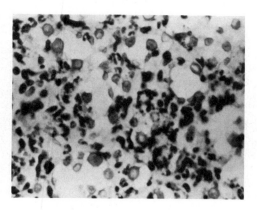

Slide 7–8.—This is a tissue section in which the cells of *C. neoformans* have been stained red. Note the size (approximately 8–10 microns) of the yeast cells. In this section the capsule is not stained; however, some of the apparently empty spaces in the tissue are (or were) filled with capsular material.

Slide 7–16. — Some laboratories do initial yeast screening with a urease test (urea agar). All *Cryptococcus* species (including *C. neoformans*) are positive in 6–72 hours, whereas *Candida albicans* and most other *Candida* species are negative. This test may also be used to aid in differentiating between *Trichophyton mentagrophytes* (positive in 2–3 days) and *T. rubrum* (negative to slightly positive after 1 week's incubation).

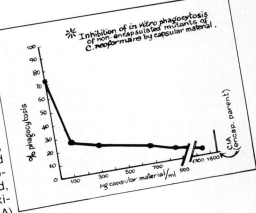

The following were discussed in greater detail in the optional portion of the chapter.

Slide 7–17. — The horizontal axis indicates 8 different strains of *Cryptococcus neoformans*. The designation C1A is the parent encapsulated strain. Strains M1–M7 are nonencapsulated mutants which were derived from the parent encapsulated strain. The vertical axis indicates the percent phagocytosis by human peripheral leukocytes. Note that the phagocytosis for the encapsulated strain is less than 20%, whereas 70–80% of the leukocytes engulfed the nonencapsulated mutants.

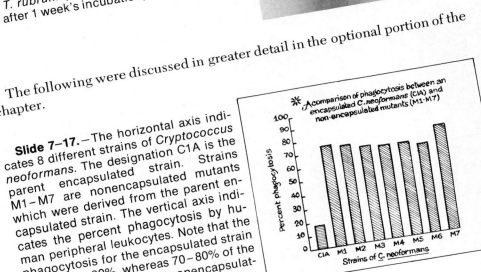

Slide 7–18. — The horizontal axis indicates increasing amounts of capsular material which were added into phagocytosis experiments. The vertical axis indicates percent phagocytosis. Note that when no capsular material was added into the phagocytic system and a nonencapsulated mutant was used, the phagocytosis was between 70% and 80%. As increasing amounts of capsular material were added into the phagocytic system containing a nonencapsulated mutant, the percent phagocytosis decreased rather rapidly. For example, when approximately 150 micrograms were added, the phagocytosis decreased to approximately 25%. The bar on the right (C1A) indicates percent phagocytosis of parent encapsulated cells.

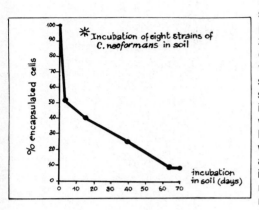

Slide 7–19.—The horizontal axis in this slide indicates incubation time in soil (days). The vertical axis indicates the percent of encapsulated cells. At time zero, when the soil was inoculated with encapsulated cells, the encapsulation was 100%. After 2–3 days' incubation in soil, 50% to 60% of the cells were encapsulated. After approximately 40 days' incubation in soil, only 25% of the cells were encapsulated. In addition to following the percent of encapsulated cells, we also recorded the size of the cells at various time intervals. These data indicated to us that *C. neoformans* may reside in soil in a relatively small and nonencapsulated state. It is this state of *C. neoformans* that is probably the infectious particle.

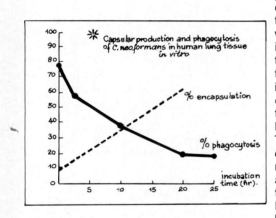

Slide 7–20.—The horizontal axis on this slide indicates incubation time in hours. The vertical axis indicates the percent phagocytosis and percent encapsulation. In these experiments we attempted to determine how much time was required for the nonencapsulated infectious particle to begin to produce the antiphagocytic capsular material after it entered the human body. From this in vitro experiment, we concluded that capsule production, and therefore inhibition of phagocytosis, required only a few hours' incubation with human tissue. This indicated to us that the body must dispose of the infectious particle rather rapidly before sufficient capsular material is produced in vivo to inhibit phagocytosis. Although it is difficult to extrapolate from in vitro to in vivo situations, we believe that the first few hours after the body is exposed to the infectious particle of *C. neoformans* are the most critical in determining if an infection will be established.

SELF-EVALUATION QUESTIONS
(Answers at end of questions)

Select the ONE best answer for each question:

1. The hallmark (outstanding characteristic) of *Cryptococcus neoformans* is
   a. _____ the method of budding
   b. _____ the size of the yeast cell
   c. _____ the formation of sporangia
   d. _____ capsule formation

2. In tissue, *Coccidioides immitis* produces
   a. _____ spherules and endospores
   b. _____ encapsulated yeast cells
   c. _____ fine, delicate hyphae
   d. _____ coarse, septate hyphae
3. Which one of the following is an intracellular parasite?
   a. _____ *Coccidioides immitis*
   b. _____ *Nocardia asteroides*
   c. _____ *Histoplasma capsulatum*
   d. _____ *Cryptococcus neoformans*
4. Cerebral infarcts are most often seen in
   a. _____ nocardiosis
   b. _____ aspergillosis
   c. _____ cryptococcosis
   d. _____ candidiasis
5. Which of the following diseases is characterized by the formation of septate, brown-colored hyphae, in vivo?
   a. _____ candidiasis
   b. _____ dematiaceous infections
   c. _____ nocardiosis
   d. _____ histoplasmosis
6. *Cryptococcus neoformans* has been found growing most often in
   a. _____ water
   b. _____ soil containing pigeon feces
   c. _____ chicken feces
   d. _____ desert soils
7. *Cryptococcus neoformans* is urease _____ (positive or negative).
8. *C. neoformans* reproduces by _____.
9. The drug of choice for cryptococcosis is _____.
10. The capsule of *C. neoformans* can be observed best in _____ preparations.
11. In suspected cases of cryptococcal meningitis the best material to culture and examine microscopically is _____.
12. Reliable skin test reagents are commercially available for the following two mycoses: _____ and _____.
13. *Nocardia* species are _____ (monomorphic or dimorphic).
14. Zygomycosis is another term for _____.
15. Clinically, cryptococcosis is most often seen causing _____.
16. Name two fungus diseases that are most often observed as hyphae growing in and around vessels: _____ and _____.

Optional Section

17. The capsule of *C. neoformans* seems to disappear when the organism is grown
   a. _____ at room temperature
   b. _____ in tissue
   c. _____ at 35 – 37 C.
   d. _____ in soil

18. Phagocytosis of *C. neoformans* is inhibited by
    a. _____ cryptococcal capsular material
    b. _____ the size of the yeast cells
    c. _____ the cell walls
    d. _____ toxins produced by the organism
19. The infectious particle of *Cryptococcus neoformans* is probably
    a. _____ the microaleuriospore
    b. _____ the tuberculate macroaleuriospore
    c. _____ a relatively small, nonencapsulated yeast
    d. _____ a chlamydospore
20. A few hours after entering the lung, the infectious particle of *Cryptococcus neoformans* begins to produce
    a. _____ hyphae
    b. _____ spores
    c. _____ toxins
    d. _____ capsular material

Answers to questions 1 to 20.

1. d
2. a
3. c
4. b
5. b
6. b
7. positive
8. budding
9. amphotericin B
10. India (China) ink

11. spinal fluid
12. coccidioidomycosis, histoplasmosis
13. monomorphic
14. phycomycosis
15. meningitis (CNS disorders)
16. aspergillosis, phycomycosis
17. d
18. a
19. c
20. d

8 / Superficial Mycoses

MANY MYCOLOGISTS categorize fungus diseases into three groups: systemic mycoses, dermatophytoses and superficial mycoses. Although these categories are useful, it is important to realize that there is a great deal of overlapping among them and that several mycoses actually fall into all three categories, e.g., candidiasis. Thus far, this book has covered some of the more important systemic and dermatophytic mycoses. This chapter presents 7 diseases which are classified as superficial mycoses—erythrasma, keratitis, otomycosis, piedras, pityriasis versicolor, trichomycosis axillaris and tinea nigra palmaris.

Superficial mycoses are fungus diseases of the outermost body layers, mainly skin, hair, ears and eyes. The dermatophytes are not classified as superficial mycoses, probably because their etiologic agents fall into a rather specialized and compact taxonomic area. Most of the superficial mycoses cause little or no tissue damage: thus, these diseases are considered primarily a cosmetic problem.

Several of the etiologic agents of superficial mycoses are now recognized as bacteria. Originally, these organisms were thought to be fungi; for that reason the diseases were named mycoses. Thus their situation is analogous to that of diseases caused by members of the Actinomycetales; i.e., it is now accepted that the etiologic agents are bacteria, but the diseases they cause are still referred to as mycoses.

ERYTHRASMA

Synonym
None.

Definition
Erythrasma is a chronic disease of the stratum corneum. The most common sites of infection are the axillary and genitocrural regions of the body. The infected area is usually very flat, is covered with scales and feels greasy. Some erythema may be noted at the edge of the lesion. The remainder of the lesion is brown to reddish. This disease develops very slowly, taking months to years for the lesions to reach several centimeters in diameter. A characteristic feature of erythrasma lesions is that they fluoresce a coral to reddish color under a Wood's or Black light.

Etiology
Corynebacterium minutissimum is now accepted as the true etiologic agent of this disease; however, the formerly accepted name, *Nocardia minutissimum,* is still in some textbooks.

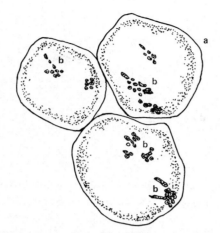

Fig 8–1. — *Corynebacterium (Nocardia) minutissimum* in skin.
A, skin cell. *B*, bacteria.

Epidemiology

Erythrasma is found worldwide, but it is especially common in tropical and subtropical areas. Many authorities believe that the etiologic agent is part of the normal skin flora of humans.

Predilections

Little is known about this subject. However, the disease occurs most frequently in young men. Some researchers have hypothesized a possible relationship between the occurrence of this disease and diabetes mellitus.

Tissue Form and Histopathology

Because this disease involves only the outermost layers of the skin, it is not worthwhile to make histological preparations for diagnostic purposes.

Direct Microscopic Examination

Obtain some skin scrapings and place them on a microscope slide. Add 1 – 2 drops of ether to defat the tissue. Pour off the ether and allow the tissue to dry. Add 1 – 2 drops of methylene blue (2 – 5 gm in 100 milliliters of 95% ethanol), press a coverslip on the preparation, heat gently and then observe microscopically with the oil immersion lens (95X). In such a preparation, *C. minutissimum* appears as small (1 micron) bacillary or diphtheroid forms. Occasionally, one may observe some fine, delicate filaments (Fig. 8 – 1).

Culture

Because it is difficult to culture this organism, culturing is rarely done. Diagnosis is usually based on clinical picture and fluorescence of lesions.

Other Laboratory Tests

None.

Therapy

In most instances erythromycin is the drug of choice (1 gram daily for 2 – 3 weeks).

KERATITIS

Synonyms

Mycotic keratitis, keratomycosis.

Definition

Any fungus infection of the cornea is called mycotic keratitis. This is usually a very serious disease which may lead to a loss of vision; for this reason, mycotic keratitis should not be classified as a superficial mycosis; it belongs with the systemic mycoses.

Etiology

At last count more than 50 species of filamentous fungi and yeast were reported as etiologic agents of mycotic keratitis, e.g., *Fusarium, Aspergillus, Curvularia, Penicillium, Cephalosporium, Candida* species. In all instances the clinical picture, disease development and therapy are the same.

Epidemiology

With only one exception, all of the etiologic agents are common soil saprophytes found worldwide. (The one exception, *Candida albicans,* is normal flora in man.) These organisms have rarely been implicated as agents of other mycoses. Most of them can be isolated from the air any place at any time.

Clinical Form

Usually, a white plaque forms on the cornea. The plaque grows very slowly (taking weeks to develop); eventually it may ulcerate. Characteristic of fungus involvement of the eye is the development of satellite lesions and endothelial plaques. Impairment of vision usually occurs.

Predilections

Because the vast majority of the numerous etiologic agents are common soil saprophytes, entrance to the eye probably follows some form of abrasion or trauma.

Tissue Form and Histopathology

Sections of infected tissue are not made, for obvious reasons, except on autopsied cases.

Direct Microscopic Examination

This procedure is of great diagnostic value. If a fungus is suspected, the ophthalmologist should remove a small piece of tissue. To culture the etiologic agent, divide the tissue into 2 pieces. Put 1 portion of tissue on a microscope slide and add 1–2 drops of 10–20% KOH. With needles, tear the tissue apart. Add a coverslip, heat gently and then press down gently on the coverslip. Examine microscopically, first at low power and then using the high dry lens.

Only one etiologic agent, *Candida albicans,* is a yeast. In KOH preparations it is seen as yeast cells with strands of pseudo-hyphae.

All of the filamentous etiologic agents appear as clear, septate hyphae in eye tissue. Because no spores or other identifying structures are formed, it is impossible to distinguish between etiologic agents in tissue. However, this procedure is extremely valuable because it shows whether a fungus is involved.

Culture

Culture tissue on Sabouraud's agar. Best results are obtained when the tissue is forced into the medium. Incubate for 1–2 weeks at room temperature. As so many fungi may be etiologic agents of this disease, specific identification procedures will not be discussed. If colonies do develop, take or send them to a mycologist for identification. Frankly, culturing and specific identification are mainly of academic interest; one needs to know only whether a fungus is involved as an etiologic agent of keratitis.

Other Laboratory Tests

None.

Therapy

In many instances, good results have been obtained with topical applications (i.e., directly on the eye) of amphotericin B, 5-fluorocytosine or 5% pimaricin. Because fungi grow slowly in tissue, they also die slowly, so it is important to continue therapy until it is certain the fungus has been killed.

OTOMYCOSIS

Synonyms

Fungus ear, mycotic otitis externa.

Definition

This is a chronic fungus infection of the outer ear and ear canal.

Etiology

Numerous filamentous fungi have been reported as etiologic agents of otomycosis. The most commonly reported organisms belong to the genera *Aspergillus*, *Mucor*, *Penicillium* and *Rhizopus*.

Epidemiology

Although this disease is found worldwide, it is more common in tropical areas. Because all of the etiologic agents are common soil saprophytes, this disease has the potential to develop any place.

Clinical Forms

Initially, the infection may be mild, resulting in only minor irritation; however, as it becomes more chronic, the infected area and surrounding ear tissue become inflamed. Pus may develop, and considerable amounts of debris may form inside the ear canal.

Many investigators doubt that there really is such a disease as otomycosis. At almost any time, fungi can be isolated from human ears, but this does not mean they are causing disease. Proof is lacking that the isolated fungi actually caused a disease process; i.e., they could be secondary, saprophytic invaders which developed as a result of a problem from another source.

Predilections

Warm temperatures and moisture increase the number of reported cases of otomycosis. Other important factors may be irritation, other ear problems and the use of irritating medications.

Tissue Form and Histopathology

This is not done. Undoubtedly this is why proof is lacking that cultured fungi actually invade healthy tissue.

Direct Microscopic Examination

Most persons think that the observation of fungi in tissue or debris, using direct microscopic examination procedures, is more important than culturing. Place material on a microscope slide, add 1–2 drops of 10% KOH and add a coverslip. Examine microscopically for the presence of hyphae.

Culture

Remove debris, scales or scrapings from the ear and culture on Sabouraud's agar at room temperature. As with mycotic keratitis, there are dozens of commonly found airborne (saprophytic) fungi that may be cultured from infected ears. For this reason, species identification will not be discussed. Take or send any cultures to a mycologist for identification if this is needed.

Other Laboratory Tests

None.

Therapy

Of primary importance is to clean and aerate the ear canal with a cotton swab saturated with Burrow's solution. Maintain this treatment for several days, along with antibacterial therapy.

PIEDRAS

Synonyms

Black and white piedra, tinea nodosa, Chignon disease, Beigel's disease.

Definition

Piedras refers to two diseases: (1) black piedra, which forms hard, dark brown to black discrete nodules on hair; (2) white piedra, which also occurs on hair but forms nodules which are not as hard and are a lighter brown.

Etiology

Black piedra is caused by *Piedraia hortai,* and white piedra is caused by *Trichosporon beigelii* (some authors prefer *T. cutaneum*). Both of these organisms are true fungi.

Epidemiology

Both diseases are found worldwide but are more common in tropical and subtropical areas. B'ack piedra occurs more commonly on scalp hairs, whereas white piedra is found primarily on facial and genital hairs. Nothing is known about the source of these diseases except that they also occur on other primates, e.g., monkeys.

Predilections

Nothing is known about this subject.

Tissue Form and Histopathology

Examinations of this type are not made because the piedras infect only hair.

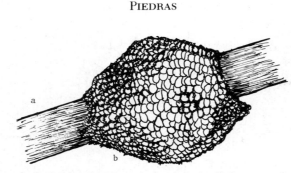

Fig 8–2.—Black piedra on hair. *A,* hair. *B,* fungus nodule.

Direct Microscopic Examination

This is the most important diagnostic procedure. Remove infected hair, place on a microscope slide with 1–2 drops of 10–20% KOH. Add a cover-slip, heat gently and press down gently. Examine microscopically under low power: (a) black piedra nodules are dark brown, discrete, almost circular, up to 1.5 millimeters in diameter. When they are broken open, asci, each containing up to 8 ascospores are seen (Fig. 8–2); (b) the nodules of white piedra are larger, softer and lighter colored than those of black piedra; the septate hyphae are not dematiaceous and tend to break into arthrospores or yeast-like cells (Fig. 8–3).

Cultures

Both of these organisms may be cultured on Sabouraud's agar at room temperature, although culturing is not necessary for diagnosis.

Colonies of *Piedraia hortai* develop very slowly, taking 2–4 weeks to reach a diameter of 1 centimeter. The colonies are dark brown and may have a metallic green tinge. They are very compact, have a raised center and are slightly fuzzy. Microscopically, one observes dematiaceous hyphae containing numerous septa.

Trichosporon beigelii cultures look very different than those of *Piedraia hortai.* They look more like yeast colonies. Such cultures are smooth to slightly wrinkled (not fuzzy) and white to tan in color. In 1–2 weeks, *T. beigelii* cultures may be 1–2 centimeters in diameter. Microscopically, one observes clear septate hyphae which may break up into individual cells.

Fig 8–3.—White piedra on hair. *A,* hair. *B,* fungus nodule.

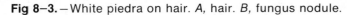
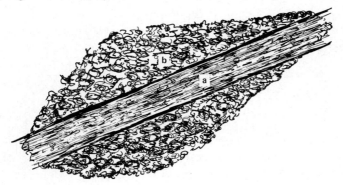

Other Laboratory Tests
None.

Therapy
Clip or shave infected areas. Treat daily with antifungal agents such as a
1:2000 solution of bichloride of mercury, 3% sulfur ointment or benzoic and
salicylic acid combinations.

PITYRIASIS VERSICOLOR

Synonyms
Liver spots, tinea versicolor, dermatomycosis furfuracea, chromophytosis.

Definition
Pityriasis versicolor is a superficial, chronic fungus infection of the horny
layer of the epidermis. Usually this disease affects the trunk of the body, although other areas may be involved. This disease causes no discomfort to the
patient, and there is no erythema or induration; essentially all that happens is
that the normal skin pigmentation is altered, resulting in a blotchy appearance. The infected areas are usually brownish. However, if scaling results, the
areas may appear lighter than the surrounding uninfected areas. In some individuals, the blotchy appearance is most noticeable after they have been in the
sun for some time. The lesions fluoresce a pale yellow under a Wood's or
black light.

Etiology
The name of the etiologic agent of this disease is *Malassezia furfur* despite
recent attempts to change it.

Epidemiology
This disease occurs worldwide and may well be one of the most common
diseases in the world. Some investigators report that its incidence in various
countries ranges from 5–50% of the population. Little is known about the
source of this organism in nature or even if it is part of man's normal flora. All
ages and sexes appear to contract the disease. Many individuals seem to be
refactory to contracting it despite intimate contact with infected persons (e.g.,
marriage partners) leading me to believe that genetic factors are important.
The highest incidence is reported in tropical areas.

Predilections
Absolutely nothing is known about this aspect of pityriasis versicolor except for my speculation about genetic factors.

Tissue Form and Histopathology
To diagnose this disease it is not necessary to examine histopathologic
preparations of skin.

Direct Microscopic Examination
Examine the patient in a dark room using a Wood's or black light. From the
areas of skin exhibiting the greatest fluorescence, scrape some of the skin into
a sterile Petri dish. Place some of the skin scrapings onto a microscope slide.
To these scrapings add either a few drops of 10% KOH, methylene blue or

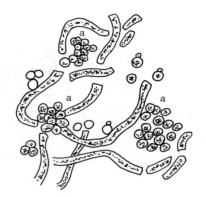

Fig 8–4. — Pityriasis versicolor in skin.
A, clusters of hyphae and yeast cells.

lactophenol cotton blue. Add a coverslip to the preparation, press down firmly and observe microscopically with a high-power lens. The organism takes up the methylene blue stain, enabling it to stand out from the skin cells. Microscopically, the organism is seen as clusters of short, angular hyphae, along with some yeast cells which are 3–8 microns in diameter (Fig. 8–4). Some authors call this a "spaghetti and meat ball" appearance.

Culture
This may be done, but it is rather difficult and not of sufficient diagnostic value to merit the trouble involved.

Other Laboratory Tests
None.

Therapy
For many years, this disease has been treated with a 10–20% aqueous solution of sodium hyposulfite applied daily. Others have success with daily applications of Whitfield's ointment or 3% salicylic acid in 70% alcohol. In some areas of the world locally manufactured vinegar is used.

Miconazole and clotrimazole are newer drugs which are said to be effective.

From my experience the treatment of choice is 1% selenium sulfide suspended in an ointment or shampoo (e.g., "Selsun Blue"). Apply undiluted, let dry and leave on overnight. Rinse off the next morning. Repeat twice at weekly intervals. Because the rate of recurrence is high (regardless of the treatment), repeat once every 6–12 months.

TRICHOMYCOSIS AXILLARIS

Synonyms
Lepothrix, trichomycosis nodosa, trichomycosis chromatica.

Definition
This disease is found only on the axillary and pubic hairs of humans. The organism grows on the hair shafts and produces greasy concretions around them. The concretions may be yellow, red or black. Eventually, hairs weaken and break off. The disease causes little discomfort to the patient.

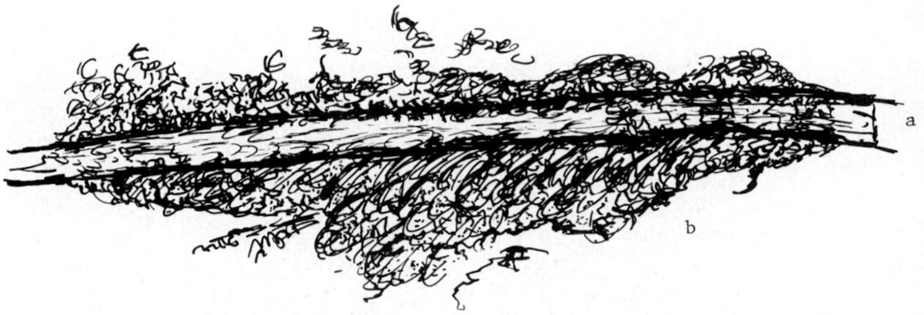

Fig 8–5.—Trichomycosis axillaris. *A*, hair. *B*, infected area.

Etiology

This is another disease originally believed to be caused by a fungus; however, it is now accepted that the true etiologic agent is the bacterium *Corynebacterium tenuis.*

Epidemiology

This disease is found worldwide, but most cases are reported from tropical or subtropical areas. It appears to be more widespread where heat and moisture favor the growth of the organism. Little is known about the source of this organism in nature or how the disease is spread.

Predilections

Little is known about this subject.

Tissue Form and Histopathology

As this organism infects hair only, one never examines histopathologic preparations.

Direct Microscopic Examination

This is an important parameter in the diagnosis of the disease. Remove some infected hair and place it on a microscope slide with 1–2 drops of 10–20% KOH. Add a coverslip, heat gently and press down on the coverslip. Examine under the low-power lens. At first, the hair shaft appears to be surrounded with greasy looking, irregular concretions (Fig. 8–5). Under higher power, fine strands or clumps of bacteria may be discernible. The bacteria are seen more readily if infected hair is smeared onto a microscope slide, stained by the gram method and examined with an oil immersion lens.

Culture

This procedure is of little value in diagnosing the disease.

Other Laboratory Tests

None.

Therapy

Hair in the infected area is shaved off. Daily applications of a 2% solution of formalin in alcohol are said to be effective. Other investigators have reported success with bichloride of mercury (1%) in 70% alcohol or a 3% sulphur ointment.

TINEA NIGRA PALMARIS

Synonyms

Keratomycosis nigricans palmaris, pityriasis nigra, microsporosis nigra.

Definition

Tinea nigra palmaris is usually seen on the palms of the hands. The dematiaceous fungus grows in or under the surface layer of the skin, causing a lesion which is dark brown to black in color. This lesion is flat, not scaly, and does not induce erythema or inflammation. The infected area looks as if the skin has been stained with a dark dye. As with most other fungus diseases, the infected area increases in size very slowly. The disease causes little or no discomfort to the patient. The most important feature of this disease is that clinicians may confuse it with skin cancer, syphilis or other serious diseases.

Etiology

This disease is caused by the dematiaceous fungus *Cladosporium werneckii.*

Epidemiology

The etiologic agent of tinea nigra palmaris is commonly found in soil throughout the world. It has been speculated that the fungus gains entrance to the superficial layers of the skin through mild trauma. Very often, this disease is seen in patients who work with their hands a great deal and are engaged in some type of agricultural occupation. Other than this, little is known about its dissemination. This disease is found most often in tropical areas such as South America and Southeast Asia.

Predilections

Almost nothing is known about why certain persons contract this disease.

Tissue Form and Histopathology

To diagnose this disease, there is little need to examine histopathological preparations. Unfortunately, such preparations are often made when a physician suspects a more serious disease. When the preparations are examined, the fungus appears in tissue as long strands of strongly septate, dematiaceous hyphae. This organism is so dematiaceous that it may readily be seen in unstained tissue sections.

Fig 8–6. — *Cladosporium werneckii* in tissue (tinea nigra palmaris).
A, skin cells. *B,* dematiaceous hypha.

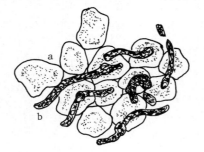

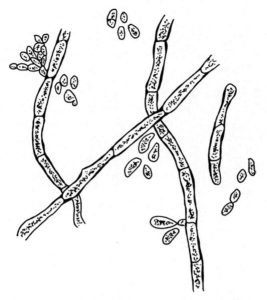

Fig 8–7. — *Cladosporium werneckii* in vitro.

Direct Microscopic Examination

This procedure is most useful in diagnosing the disease. Place some skin scrapings on a microscope slide, add 1–2 drops of 10–20% KOH, add a coverslip and heat gently. Press down firmly on the coverslip and examine the preparation under low power. The organism is seen as septate, dematiaceous strands of hyphae. The outstanding feature of this organism is that the hyphae are strongly dematiaceous. Also, some of the hyphae contain numerous chlamydospores (Fig. 8–6).

Culture

To reduce the possibility of bacterial contamination from the skin, the infected area should first be decontaminated with 70% alcohol. Then, gently scrape off some of the skin and place it onto Sabouraud's agar and, with a stiff inoculation needle, force some of the skin scrapings into the medium. Incubate at room temperature to 30 C. In 7–10 days, dark colonies will form. At first these colonies will look yeast-like. After an additional 1–2 weeks' incubation, the culture becomes 1–2 centimeters in diameter, and the fungus begins to produce some fluffy-looking, aerial hyphae. Remove some of the fungus from the culture and examine it microscopically. In such preparations it is possible to observe strongly septate, dematiaceous hyphae, which may produce dark-colored spores that give the appearance of yeast cells (Fig. 8–7).

Other Laboratory Tests

None.

Therapy

Several of the recommended treatments for this disease are 3% sulphur and 2% salicylic acid, tincture of iodine or weak Whitfield's ointment. Actually, any type of treatment that tends to sluff the outer layers of skin and has a mild fungicidal effect is of value.

Slides

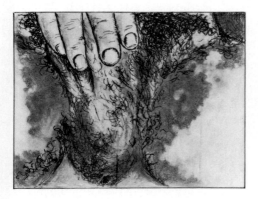

Slide 8–1.—This is a patient with erythrasma. The lesion is relatively flat, not erythematous at the edge, and brown throughout. This lesion took several months to develop to this size.

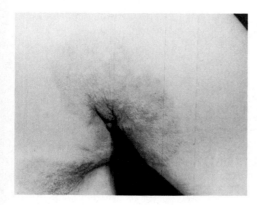

Slide 8–2.—This is an excellent example of the red lesion form of erythrasma.

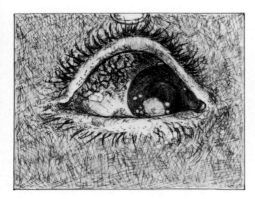

Slide 8–3.—This is a rather typical case of mycotic keratitis. The patient reported that several months previously some foreign matter had lodged in his eye.

Slide 8–4.—In this case of mycotic keratitis the lesion is not as obvious; however, at the edge of the cornea one gets a hint of the formation of satellite lesions, which, to the ophthalmologist, is one of the most important diagnostic features of fungus infections of the eye. Scrapings from this eye were examined in KOH preparations, and septate hyphae were observed. Additional material was cultured, and the etiologic agent was identified as a *Fusarium.* The patient was given topical treatment with amphotericin B and responded in a satisfactory fashion.

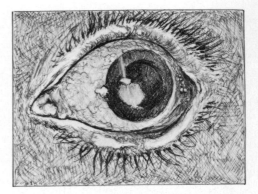

Slide 8–5.—This is what one sees in cases of mycotic keratitis when infected tissue is observed microscopically under direct examination procedures. Note the presence of hyphae (A, B). In this photograph, it is difficult to determine whether the hyphae are septate or coenocytic. This particular organism was cultured on Sabouraud's medium and identified as an *Aspergillus* species.

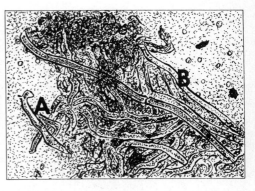

Slide 8–6.—This, like the previous slide, is a direct examination preparation from a case of mycotic keratitis. Note the abundance of clear, septate hyphae (A, B). When structures of this nature are observed, there is no doubt that the etiologic agent is a fungus.

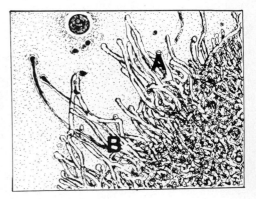

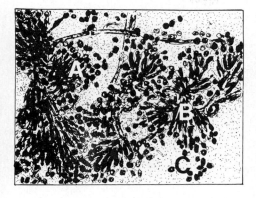

Slide 8–7.—The *Penicillium* organism first gained medical fame as the producer of the antibiotic penicillin; however, it has been known for many years that there are a myriad of *Penicillium* species, and some of them have been implicated occasionally as the etiologic agents of human disease. This organism has septate hyphae which are not particularly characteristic; however, note the manner in which the spores are borne. Throughout this photograph are numerous flask-like structures held together in clusters (A, B). The grouping of these clusters is frequently referred to as "brushes," and it is upon such structures that the small spores are borne. A few spores (C) can be seen in this photograph on the end of these flask-like structures (sterigma) and floating free in the preparation. *Penicillium* species are implicated in otomycosis and mycotic keratitis.

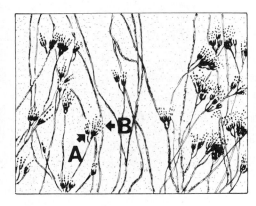

Slide 8–8.—This is a photomicrograph of another species of *Penicillium*. Here the brushes (A) with a few spores (B) attached to them can be seen more clearly.

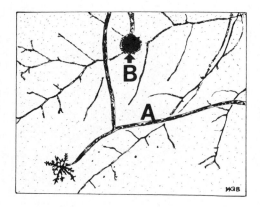

Slide 8–9.—This is the fungus *Rhizopus,* another etiologic agent of otomycosis and mycotic keratitis. There are 3 important features of species found in the genus *Rhizopus,* and all 3 of these can be observed in this picture: The hyphae (A) are relatively large (8–10 microns in diameter) and are coenocytic; the larger, spherical, dark blue structure in this photograph is a sporangium (B), and, under high magnification, one would see that it contains dozens of spores (sporangiospores); at the end of a piece of hypha, one can see a mass of finger-like projections, the so-called rhizoids from which the genus name is derived. The purpose of the rhizoids is probably to hold the fungus to the substrate and absorb nutrients.

Slide 8–10.—This fungus, *Fusarium,* is another etiologic agent of otomycosis and mycotic keratitis. This organism produces clear septate hyphae which are not particularly characteristic. Looking closer at this slide, one sees that *Fusarium* produces 2 types of spores: microconidia (A), which are the small, ovoid spores; and macroconidia (B), which are the larger, septate, new-moon-shaped spores.

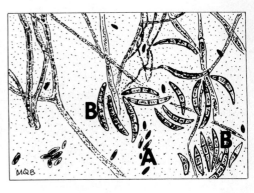

Slide 8–11.—This is a typical picture of an *Aspergillus* species. This fungus produces clear septate hyphae. Note the way the spores are borne. On the ends of the specialized pieces of hyphae (conidiophores) (A) is a swollen tip (vesicle) (B). On these vesicles, phialides (or sterigma) are present, and long strands of small spores (C) are borne at the end of the sterigma. *Aspergillus* species cause otomycosis, mycotic keratitis and aspergillosis.

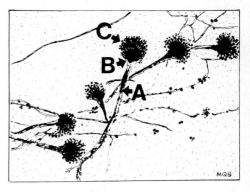

Slide 8–12.—This is a low-magnification photograph of hair with black piedra. Note the discrete nodules surrounding the hair shafts (A, B).

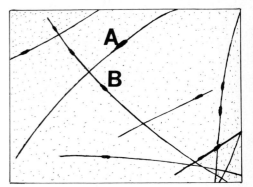

Slide 8–13.—This is a higher magnification photograph of hair with black piedra. The lesion (A) is very discrete, surrounds the hair shaft and is dark brown. Eventually the fungus may weaken the hair shaft to the extent that the hair breaks off.

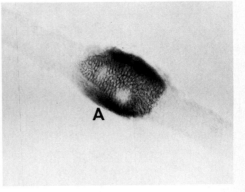

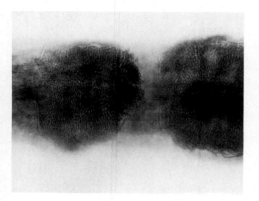

Slide 8–14. — This is a still higher magnification of hair infected with *Piedraia hortai.* Close observation reveals that the nodule appears to be composed of hundreds of spherical cells. These cells are the asci, which contain ascospores. Such structures can be seen more clearly when one places infected hair in 1–2 drops of 10–20% KOH on a microscope slide, adds a coverslip, heats the preparation gently and then presses down very firmly on the coverslip. In such preparations the piedra nodules break open, and one sees many individual asci containing ascospores and, occasionally, groups of ascospores which have been squeezed out of individual asci.

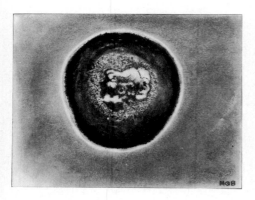

Slide 8–15. — This is a culture of the fungus *Piedraia hortai.* This fungus was cultured on Sabouraud's medium and incubated at room temperature. It normally takes 4–6 weeks' incubation for a colony to reach this size. The gross features of this colony are that it is slow-growing, is heaped up in the center, is a dark brown-black to metallic green and is surrounded by a clear ring where the young growing mycelium has not yet produced the dark pigment. Microscopically, there are few characteristic features: the fungus produces dematiaceous hyphae which may contain numerous chlamydospores. No characteristic spores are produced.

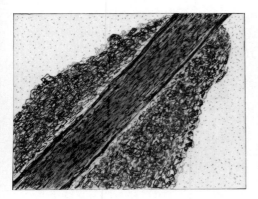

Slide 8–16. — In this picture we see hair infected with white piedra *(Trichosporon beigelii).* Note that, when this nodule is compared with that seen in black piedra, it is not as discrete and lacks the dark coloration. Additionally, this fungus does not produce ascospores. When cultured on Sabouraud's agar and incubated for 2–4 weeks at room temperature, this fungus produces a rough, membranous, white to light tan colony. Microscopically, the organism produces no characteristic spores. (Slides 8–15 and 8–16 courtesy of E. S. Beneke, from *Human Mycoses,* 1968.)

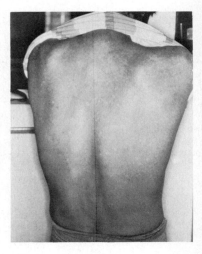

Slide 8–17. — Note the numerous, relatively small areas of hypopigmentation. This is pityriasis versicolor.

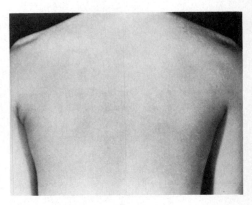

Slide 8–18. — This also is pityriasis versicolor. Note the larger area of hypopigmentation in the center. In this disease there is no erythema, the infected areas are not elevated, and, aside from some itching the patient feels no discomfort.

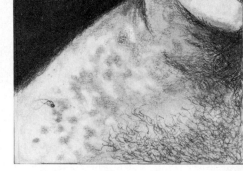

Slide 8–19. — This is a patient with pityriasis versicolor on the right shoulder. Again, note the blotchiness of the skin pigmentation.

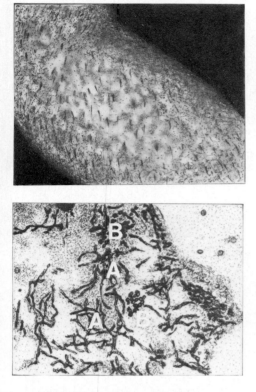

Slide 8–20.—This slide shows a patient infected with pityriasis versicolor being observed under an ultraviolet, Wood's or black light. Note the speckled appearance of the skin.

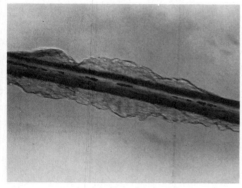

Slide 8–21.—This is a photomicrograph of skin infected with *Malassezia furfur*. Note that in vivo this organism produces clusters or clumps of rather short hyphae (A) and spherical yeast cells (B). Some authors refer to this overall picture as "spaghetti and meatballs."

Slide 8–22.—This is a close-up photograph of hair with trichomycosis. Note that the hairs are surrounded by greasy concretions. In this particular case, the concretions are light colored; however, in some cases they are red or black. Eventually the organism weakens the hair shaft to the point where it may break off.

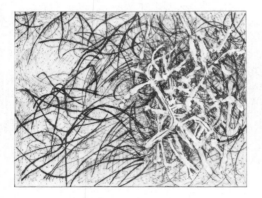

Slide 8–23.—This is a low-power photomicrograph of hair with trichomycosis. Note that a large portion of the hair shaft is surrounded by greasy-looking, irregular concretions. This disease is caused by a bacterium. If one wishes to observe the etiologic agent microscopically, it is recommended that a smear from infected hairs be made onto a microscope slide and stained, with the gram method. Observe such preparations using the oil immersion lens of the microscope.

Slide 8–24.—This is a photograph of tissue prepared for direct examination with 10% KOH. Throughout the field one can readily observe strongly septate dematiaceous hyphae (A,B). Note: No coloring agent has been added to this slide; the dark brown color is produced in the fungus. This is how the etiologic agent of tinea nigra palmaris appears in tissue. The fungal cells in this preparation which appear to be more rounded are chlamydospores. It is not uncommon to see such structures in tinea nigra palmaris.

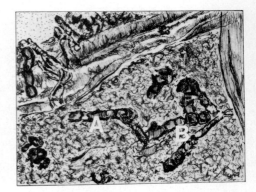

Tinea nigra palmaris is strictly superficial; i.e., it does not have systemic manifestations. However, certain dematiaceous fungi can cause subcutaneous or brain abscesses. In these instances, internal organs are involved. As yet, no one has come up with a suitable name for these diseases; however, they are definitely not referred to as tinea nigra palmaris. When there is systemic involvement, one observes, in KOH preparations, elements which appear identical to those seen in Slide 8–24.

SELF-EVALUATION QUESTIONS
(Answers at end of questions)

Check the ONE correct answer for each question:

1. Several of the etiologic agents of superficial mycoses are
   a. _____ viruses
   b. _____ bacteria
   c. _____ yeast
   d. _____ dimorphic fungi
2. Erythrasma is usually seen in which of the following body regions or tissues?
   a. _____ palms
   b. _____ scalp
   c. _____ nails
   d. _____ genitocrural region
3. One yeast reported to cause mycotic keratitis is
   a. _____ *Candida albicans*
   b. _____ *Cryptococcus neoformans*
   c. _____ *Candida keratitis*
   d. _____ *Saccharomyces species*
4. The most common causes of mycotic keratitis is (are)
   a. _____ filamentous fungi
   b. _____ yeast
   c. _____ dematiaceous fungi
   d. _____ coenocytic fungi
5. Most of the etiologic agents of otomycosis are
   a. _____ yeast

    b. _____ dermatophytes

    c. _____ systemic fungal pathogens

    d. _____ airborne fungi

6. The disease which presents as black discrete nodules on hair is

    a. _____ erythrasma

    b. _____ trichomycosis axillaris

    c. _____ white piedra

    d. _____ black piedra

7. Which of the following fungi form asci (and ascospores) in vivo?

    a. _____ *Cladosporium werneckii*

    b. _____ *Piedraia hortai*

    c. _____ *Candida albicans*

    d. _____ *Trichosporon beigelii*

8. Grossly, the colonies of *Piedraia hortai* are

    a. _____ white and fluffy

    b. _____ yeast-like

    c. _____ dark brown

    d. _____ bacterial looking

9. In direct microscopic examination preparations of hair infected with *Corynebacterium tenuis* one observes

    a. _____ bacteria

    b. _____ yeast

    c. _____ clear, septate hyphae

    d. _____ dematiaceous hyphae

10. In direct microscopic examination preparations of skin infected with *Cladosporium werneckii* one observes

    a. _____ bacteria

    b. _____ yeast

    c. _____ clear, septate hyphae

    d. _____ dematiaceous hyphae

For the following questions, fill in the blanks:

11. The most commonly occurring superficial mycosis is _____ _____.

12. *Malassezia furfur* is the etiologic agent of _____ _____.

13. Yellow, red or black concretions on hair are seen in the disease _____ _____.

14. The tragedy of tinea nigra palmaris is that it may be mistaken for _____, _____ or _____.

15. A cause of mycotic keratitis, which is also a part of man's normal flora is the organism _____ _____.

16. Superficial mycoses are "fungus" diseases of the outmost body layers, mainly, _____, _____, _____ and _____.

17. A flat, dark, nonerythematous lesion seen on the hand may be _____ _____.

18. An agent of otomycosis which produces "brushes" in culture is _____.

19. The superficial mycosis that produces a greasy concretion on hair is

_____   _____.

20. An etiologic agent of otomycosis which produces both microconidia and macroconidia is _____.

Answers to questions 1–20.

1. b	11. pityriasis versicolor
2. d	12. pityriasis versicolor
3. a	13. trichomycosis axillaris
4. a	14. skin cancer, syphilis, other serious diseases
5. d	15. *Candida albicans*
6. d	16. skin, hair, ear, eyes
7. b	17. tinea nigra palmaris
8. c	18. *Penicillium*
9. a	19. trichomycosis axillaris
10. d	20. *Fusarium*

9 / Self-Evaluation Exercise

SLIDE UNKNOWNS FROM ALL CHAPTERS

You have read this book and so reached the "expert" level in medical mycology. Now take the self-evaluation exercise consisting of 20 unknown slides. Study the slides carefully, read the following comments and answer the questions. Answers are given at the end of the chapter.

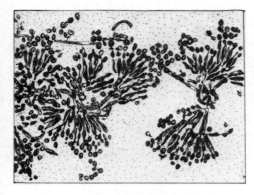

Slide 9–1. — This is a microculture of a rather common air contaminant. In a few rare instances, some of the species belonging to this genus have been reported to cause human disease. Note that the spores seem to develop on brushes. One member of this genus is famous for the production of the first antibiotic. Name the genus.

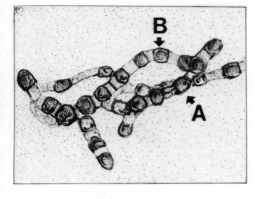

Slide 9–2. — This is a photomicrograph of a very infectious fungus. In nature, this organism resides in soil in desert areas. The spores are the infectious particles (A, B). Name the spores and the fungus.

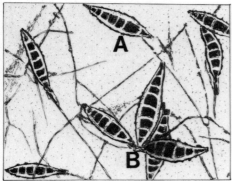

Slide 9–3. — This is a photomicrograph of a fungus isolated from a dermatophytic skin lesion. Grossly, the culture was white on the top and a bright canary color on the underside. The macroaleuriospores (A, B) usually have 8 – 12 septa and thick rough walls, and the ends are narrowed. Name the organism.

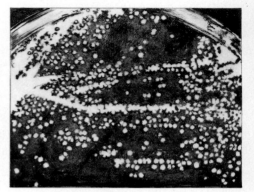

Slide 9–4. — This is a culture of a monomorphic, nonencapsulated, common pathogenic yeast. This should be enough information to name the genus. Additionally, name one important identification medium that can be used to identify the most notable species in this genus.

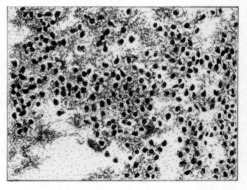

Slide 9–5. — This picture shows a patient who has had this fungus disease for several years. The infected area has many draining sinus tracts from which granules were obtained. Name the disease.

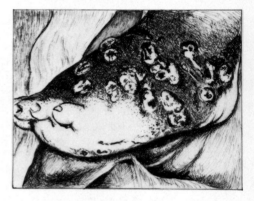

Slide 9–6. — This is a section of adrenal tissue heavily infected with a relatively small, nonencapsulated, intracellular yeast. Name the disease. Is the etiologic agent monomorphic or dimorphic?

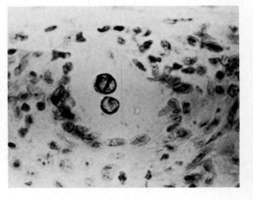

Slide 9–7. — This is a photomicrograph of a stained pathology slide; however, the fungal elements in the middle of the slide would be brown even in unstained preparations. Note that this cluster of fungal elements shows neither hyphal formation nor yeast cells. Closer examination of the structures would indicate that they seem to divide by splitting down the middle. What is the name of these fungal elements?

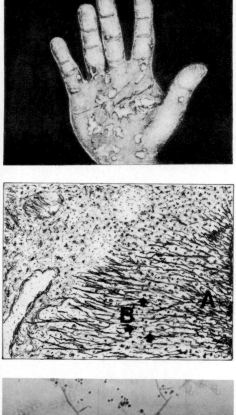

Slide 9–8.—This is the hand of a patient who was treated for a ringworm infection. This reaction is a result of an allergy to the drug he was receiving. Name the antibiotic.

Slide 9–9.—This is a photomicrograph of a section of infected esophagus stained with PAS. The pink elements are the fungus (A). Although the fungus appears to be dividing exclusively by hyphal formation, if one looks more closely it is possible to see numerous yeast cells mixed in with the hyphae (B). Name the disease.

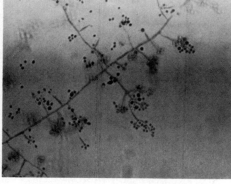

Slide 9–10.—This is a photomicrograph of a human pathogen that was cultured on Sabouraud's agar medium at room temperature. When the culture was transferred to brain-heart infusion agar medium and incubated at 35 C, long, slender yeast cells were seen microscopically. Name the organism.

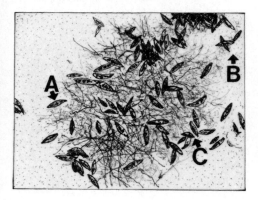

Slide 9–11.—This is a photomicrograph of a fungus isolated from soil. This organism is a dermatophyte commonly isolated from soil, but occasionally it causes such human diseases as tinea barbae. The aleuriospores in this culture have thin walls, are spindle-shaped and typically contain 2–5 septa (A, B, C). Name the organism.

Slide 9–12.—This patient has a fungus disease which originated on the hand and then spread up the lymph channels of the arm. A dimorphic fungus was isolated. Name the disease.

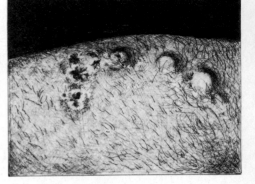

Slide 9–13.—This is a methenamine silver stain (GMS) of infected tissue. Note the numerous, dark-colored yeast cells, 10–15 microns in diameter. Name the disease. If this is not enough information, go on to the next slide.

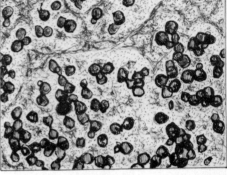

Slide 9–14.—This is a higher magnification of the yeast cells seen in Slide 9–13. Note how one of the yeast cells is dividing (A). The dividing yeast cell is forming a very broad base at the neck of the blastospore. Name the specific organism.

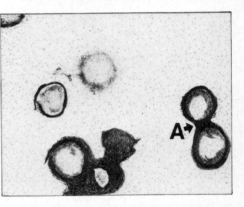

Slide 9–15.—A dermatophyte has been isolated from a skin lesion. The surface of the colony is white and fluffy, while the underside is dark yellow, almost brown. Microscopically, the organism is forming numerous microaleuriospores. One of 2 organisms is suspected, so the hair penetration test is performed. In this slide, we see the hair which has been incubated with this fungus for 2–3 weeks. Name the organism.

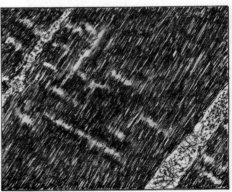

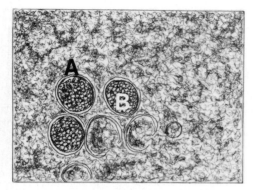

Slide 9–16.—This is tissue removed from a mouse which was inoculated with an arthrospore suspension of a fungus which causes a systemic disease. Look closely at the slide; toward the middle, note the spherical structures (20–30 microns in diameter) containing numerous spores (A, B). Name the disease.

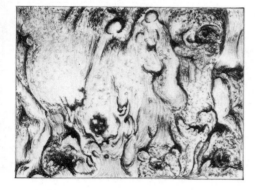

Slide 9–17.—This is a piece of human ileum removed from a patient with a fatal fungus disease. The etiologic agent was a monomorphic, nonencapsulated yeast. On chlamydospore agar this organism formed yeast cells, pseudo-hyphae and chlamydospores. Name the genus and species.

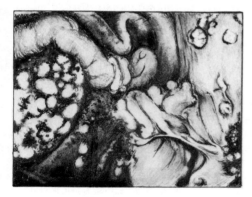

Slide 9–18.—This shows the internal organs of a guinea pig inoculated with a member of the Actinomycetales. The organism was partially acid-fast; the culture was yellow and had an earthy odor. Name the disease.

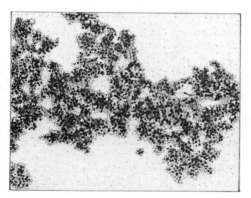

Slide 9–19.—This is a photomicrograph of a 37 C culture of a dimorphic fungal pathogen. These yeast cells are very small, and all of them appear spherical. When this organism was cultured on Sabouraud's medium and incubated at room temperature for 2–3 weeks, a fluffy, white mycelial culture developed, which, microscopically, contained tuberculate macroaleuriospores. There should be no question of the name of this organism.